Finding Calm for
the Expectant Mom

ALSO BY ALICE D. DOMAR, Ph.D.

HEALING MIND, HEALTHY WOMAN:
Using the Mind–Body Connection to
Manage Stress and Take Control of Your Life

SIX STEPS TO INCREASED FERTILITY:
An Integrated Medical and Mind/Body
Program to Promote Conception (coauthor)

SELF-NURTURE:
Learning to Care for Yourself
as Effectively as You Care for Everyone Else

CONQUERING INFERTILITY:
Dr. Alice Domar's Mind/Body Guide to
Enhancing Fertility and Coping with Infertility

BE HAPPY WITHOUT BEING PERFECT:
How to Worry Less and Enjoy Life More

LIVE A LITTLE!
Breaking the Rules Won't Break Your Health
(with Dr. Susan Love)

Finding Calm

FOR THE

Expectant Mom

Tools for Reducing Stress, Anxiety,
and Mood Swings During
Your Pregnancy

✌

ALICE D. DOMAR, Ph.D.,
and SHEILA CURRY OAKES

A TarcherPerigee Book

tarcherperigee

An imprint of Penguin Random House LLC
375 Hudson Street
New York, New York 10014

Tarcher and Perigee are registered trademarks, and the colophon is a
trademark of Penguin Random House LLC.

Most TarcherPerigee books are available at special quantity discounts for
bulk purchase for sales promotions, premiums, fund-raising, and educational
needs. Special books or book excerpts also can be created to fit specific
needs. For details, write: Special.Markets@penguinrandomhouse.com.

Library of Congress Cataloging-in-Publication Data

Names: Domar, Alice D., author. | Curry Oakes, Sheila, author.
Title: Finding calm for the expectant mom : tools for reducing stress,
anxiety, and mood swings during your pregnancy /
Alice D. Domar, PhD, with Sheila Curry Oakes.
Description: New York, New York : TarcherPerigee, [2016]
Identifiers: LCCN 2016004892 | ISBN 9780399173134 (paperback)
Subjects: LCSH: Pregnancy—Popular works. | Childbirth—Popular works. |
Women—Health and hygiene. | Stress management for women. |
BISAC: HEALTH & FITNESS / Pregnancy & Childbirth. |
SELF-HELP / Stress Management. |
HEALTH & FITNESS / Women's Health.
Classification: LCC RG525 .D653 2016 | DDC 618.2—dc23

Printed in the United States of America
1   3   5   7   9   10   8   6   4   2

Book design by Katy Riegel

To Sarah and Katie,

the fantastic outcomes of

my times as an expectant mom.

You have brought me more joy than

I ever thought possible.

LYM,
Mom

❧

In memory of Henry Dreher,

who introduced me to the

joy and meaning of writing.

Contents

Foreword

As an obstetrician, I am well aware that pregnancy has both joys and trials. The problem is that many of my patients expect the joys but not the trials. Now, Ali Domar has provided this beautifully written and practical guide that will help women see a more realistic view of both sides of pregnancy and learn some simple yet highly effective techniques to cope with the mood changes and anxiety that can come with even the healthiest of pregnancies. My favorite part is the appendix of mind/body resources, "The Calm Mom-to-Be—Mind/Body Techniques to Reduce Stress and Anxiety." I found myself applying some of the techniques to stressful areas of my own life: stop, breathe, reflect, and choose. The stories and lessons we learn from Domar are filled with her particular brand of experience, wisdom, warmth, and humor. If you've ever been lucky enough to hear Dr. Domar speak, you'll hear her voice throughout the book. Having this trusted voice to help guide women through pregnancy brings calm to me!

Hope A. Ricciotti, M.D.
Chair, Department of Obstetrics and Gynecology,
Beth Israel Deaconess Medical Center, Harvard Medical School

Introduction

THINK ABOUT THE words many of us use to describe pregnancy. "Miraculous." "Joyful." "Blissful." "Awe inspiring." "Amazing." "Perfect." "Exciting." "Glowing." "A dream come true." "A blessing." "The most incredible experience of a woman's life." If this is the way you are feeling all the time, you don't need this book. But if you also have your share of challenging moments, read on!

These were some of the words that were flying around in the mind of Liv, one of my patients, who got pregnant not long after she began seeing me for counseling.

"The test was positive—I'm pregnant!" she gushed on the phone just minutes after receiving her results. "Now that I'm pregnant, my life is perfect! I have everything I've ever wanted. My dream has come true! I don't need counseling anymore."

I had my doubts. But I didn't want to rain on Liv's

parade, so I congratulated her and told her to call me if she changed her mind. "I'm always here for you," I said. Liv had become pregnant after about six months of trying. During that time, she had been pretty miserable; she wanted so much to become a mother, and she felt terribly frustrated by how long it had taken her to conceive. She struggled with feelings of sadness, worry, and guilt. Arguments between her and her husband sprang up more frequently than they had before, and Liv had started to lose interest in her career.

I was thrilled for Liv; I knew how deeply she yearned for a baby. But I also worried about her a bit. Pregnancy is indeed an amazing, miraculous, exciting experience. But it is also a momentous physical and emotional challenge that many first-time mothers—like Liv—underestimate.

In a Word

Words most commonly associated with pregnancy, according to legend:

Radiant
Peaceful
Glowing
Contented
Serene
Fulfilled
Madonna
Feminine
Happy
Womanly

Words most commonly associated with pregnancy, according to Google:

Tired	*Stretch marks*
Dizzy	*Worry*
Painful	*Expensive*
Big	*Uncomfortable*
Morning sickness	*Swelling*

It didn't surprise me a few weeks later when Liv called to make an appointment to see me. Her pregnancy was progressing normally, but she didn't feel amazing, awesome, or perfect. She felt physically tapped out by morning sickness and fatigue. Her emotions confused her; instead of feeling joyful and satisfied, she felt cheerless and distressed, miserable rather than blissful. Arguments between her and her husband were occurring even more frequently than before.

We ended up meeting every few weeks for the rest of her pregnancy, in part because she was so embarrassed to be finding pregnancy so difficult and because she felt she had nobody else to talk to about it. She didn't feel comfortable unloading on her husband, because he had suffered alongside her during the months of trying. Her friends and family who had supported her during that time expressed confusion when she complained about pregnancy: Wasn't it what she had wanted for so long? Shouldn't she be happy? What did she have to complain about?

Liv wanted to be happy, and in fact, in an intellectual sense, she was completely thrilled to be pregnant. But her emotional side was flabbergasted by the physical and psychological demands of pregnancy. And she was shocked that pregnancy hadn't erased the anxieties, guilt, and expectations that she'd experienced while trying to conceive.

The story ends happily. Liv made it through her pregnancy and had an easy delivery. Recently, she e-mailed me a photograph of her gorgeous baby, along with a note telling me that she's feeling good. But she still marvels at how unhappy she was during her pregnancy. Like so many women, Liv was completely caught off guard by the difference between the fantasy and the reality of pregnancy.

As girls and women, we buy into our culture's pregnancy fantasy. We assume it's true when we hear pregnancy described as "amazing" and "awesome" and "joyful." Then, when we conceive, we learn the reality: that pregnancy has lots of ups and downs. It can be a long, hard journey that can be physically burdensome and emotionally challenging while at the same time feeling miraculous and exciting.

Real-life pregnancy may not always be blissful, and that catches a lot of women off guard. Instead of feeling radiant, they are nauseated. Instead of feeling joyful, they're upset that their jeans are so tight. Instead of feeling elated, they're anxious. And instead of feeling perfect, they feel guilty, blaming themselves for not living up to our culture's expectations—and their own—of how a pregnant woman *should* feel.

I want to change all that, which is why I wrote *Finding Calm for the Expectant Mom*. I want pregnant women to understand that the words our culture uses to describe pregnancy cover only part of the true experience of conceiving, carrying, and delivering a baby. Yes, pregnancy is "wonderful" and "miraculous" and "amazing" and "blissful." But it's also "tiring" and "painful" and "boring" and "scary."

If you're pregnant and you're feeling anxious, blue, exhausted, disappointed, or conflicted, here's the word I would use to describe you: "normal." It's okay to feel *all* of these feelings. It's okay to feel blissful one minute and depressed the next. That's exactly how pregnancy is supposed to feel.

When my patient Liv came to see me during her pregnancy, I focused on helping her realign her expectations about pregnancy. Our work together helped her understand and accept that all kinds of feelings—positive and negative—are a normal part of the pregnant woman's psychological experience.

Finding Calm for the Expectant Mom explains, in book form, all of the ground that Liv and I (and all of my many pregnant patients) cover during our weekly therapy sessions. For ease of writing, I have used the term "he" throughout this book to refer to the pregnant woman's partner. However, almost everything in the book can and is meant to apply to a female partner as well. If you have no partner, please ignore everything that is said about one's partner, both the good and bad. If the situation is applicable to a family member or friend, please use that concept. Also, I use the term "obstetrician" (OB) to refer to one's health-care practitioner; this is intended to include nurse-midwives, family practice physicians, nurse practitioners, physician assistants, and other health-care providers. In this book, you will learn a variety of strategies and tools that will help you enjoy the good parts of your pregnancy, cope successfully with the physical and emotional challenges, and discover how to feel happier during pregnancy and beyond.

Finding Calm for the Expectant Mom

Chapter 1

Am I Crazy, or Am I Just Pregnant?

You're pregnant! Most people are probably telling you "Congratulations!" "How exciting!" "How thrilling!" You may feel thrilled and excited but likely also worried, nauseated, and a whole host of other physical and emotional symptoms—some of which you expected, but others of which, I assume, caught you by surprise. You are probably also coming to realize that being pregnant carries with it responsibilities and expectations—maybe more than you anticipated. Of course, you want to do whatever is in your power to ensure the health and well-being of your baby. But some of those expectations can weigh heavily on you, and it may be a surprise how physically and psychologically challenging pregnancy can be.

No one really talks about how most pregnancies are not

1

spent being blissfully happy or symptom-free. In fact, you've probably heard it a million times: Pregnant women *glow*. They are so radiant, so breathtakingly gorgeous, so bursting with feminine allure and blooming loveliness that the media can't help but shout about it. And shout they do. When celebrities are pregnant, they seem to sail through the nine months without morning sickness or significant weight gain and are back in their skinny jeans before you know it. And oh, how they *glow*!

I could fill this book with the claims people make about the glow of pregnancy. It is an idea that is entrenched in our pregnancy mythology. It is something we all want to believe; wouldn't it be wonderful to be radiant for nine months? Except for one thing: It's simply not true. The "glow" of pregnancy is a complete myth. Sure, some of us shine a bit when we're expecting a baby. But to expect to glow for forty weeks is unrealistic. (Listen to what Jessica Simpson had to say about this: "People always say that pregnant women have a glow. And I say it's because you're sweating to death.") The reality of pregnancy is not so glittery or glamorous. The normal physical and emotional symptoms of pregnancy—especially in the first trimester—are often the polar opposite of "glowing."

I'll tell you a story that illustrates this perfectly. As the founder and director of a unique health-care organization, the Domar Centers for Mind/Body Health, I work alongside a staff of integrative care providers—psychologists, acupuncturists, nutritionists, yoga teachers, and others—to help patients tend to their physical and emotional health. We provide a wide range of services, including the Mind/Body Program for Infertility, which teaches relaxation strategies and stress-management skills while offering support for women who are struggling to conceive.

At the beginning and the end of each ten-week program, each patient completes an assessment designed to measure symptoms of depression. We use it to compare depression symptoms in it our patients at the start and the end of our programs. Almost always, we discover that women feel far less depressed at the conclusion of our programs. Well, this is the case for *nearly* every woman who participates in our programs—with one exception: newly pregnant women. When they take the questionnaire, their scores for depressive symptoms are often off the charts.

The interesting thing is, they don't score high on the depression scale because women in their first trimester all feel depressed about being pregnant. On the contrary, they are thrilled about it. So why do they score so high on depressive symptoms? Well, when you compare some of the most common symptoms of pregnancy with symptoms of depression, you really can't tell the difference between the two. And we're talking about the *normal* symptoms of pregnancy.

Pregnancy	Depression
Worry about the future	Worry about the future
Loss of energy	Loss of energy
Changes in sleeping patterns	Changes in sleeping patterns
Changes in appetite	Changes in appetite
Difficulty concentrating	Difficulty concentrating
Tiredness or fatigue	Tiredness or fatigue
Loss of interest in sex	Loss of interest in sex

It comes down to this: The physical and emotional symptoms of the first trimester can be so similar to those of depression that it's hard to find a newly pregnant woman who *doesn't* appear at least somewhat depressed. Or at least feel yucky. Even if she is eagerly looking forward to being a mother, she can be sad, anxious, or worried about her pregnancy or impending motherhood.

Then, on top of it all, pregnant women often feel *guilty* because they don't feel fabulous. Or they feel guilty because they do. And they feel guilty if they voice a complaint about being pregnant—especially if they have worked hard to become pregnant. If others put a positive spin on pregnancy, they feel badly if they don't match their enthusiasm. Or, if others put a negative spin on pregnancy, it's easy to go down the negative rabbit hole and be upset by horror stories or see any of their own symptoms or feelings as largely negative. Or they can feel completely confused because they are trying to balance the challenges of physical symptoms with the happiness they are feeling or, conversely, feel perfectly fine physically but strangely ambivalent about having a baby. Pregnancy emotions can range from giddy one moment to depleted the next.

Tess, mom of an eight-month-old, expresses what many women feel: "The first trimester was a mix of emotions. My husband and I were on the fence about having kids, so it was a little scary that I was pregnant. At around six or eight weeks, I thought, 'This is a terrible idea,' but at the same time I was really happy . . . and anxious, scared, and excited. Everything I could be feeling—I did! By the second trimester, people were telling me 'don't be stressed,' but trying *not* to be stressed is so *stressful*!"

Feeling anxious, moody, and exhausted during pregnancy is *normal*. So is not feeling anxious, moody, and exhausted. There is no one right way to feel. But the fantasy of contentedly rubbing our growing bellies is only partially true. You can in fact be maternal to the max while simultaneously resenting how nauseated and tired you are feeling. Feeling happy and overwhelmed at the same time is the definition of a normal pregnancy.

⚘

Normal Pregnancy Perspectives

"I'm not in it to be pregnant; I'm in it for the baby!"

"I am surprised by how much I loved being pregnant. I loved it."

"No one told me it would be this uncomfortable."

"I don't want to be pregnant again, but I enjoyed giving birth."

"I was a little sad that the pregnancy was over."

Surprising Symptoms

During pregnancy—especially the first months—you are far more likely to be gagging than glowing. In fact, it's common to feel all kinds of surprising physical and emotional symptoms. Even if you are totally thrilled to be pregnant, you're likely to start your nine-month journey experiencing uncomfortable symptoms, including fatigue, nausea, breast tenderness, bloating, insomnia, gassiness, and aversions to certain odors. And until it happens to you—until you start feeling the physical and emotional effects of pregnancy—you simply can't imagine what it feels like, even if you've watched friends and family members go through it. Many of my patients, in anticipation of getting pregnant, read all sorts of well-meaning but unrealistic books and blogs about pregnancy. Many of these portray picture-perfect pregnancies. After all, who wants to read about vomiting and hemorrhoids? Swelling and sleeplessness? Because of the unrealistic portrayal of pregnancy, I find myself having the same conversation week after week. A pregnant patient comes in, feeling guilty about not feeling great; I reassure her that her feelings are totally normal, which of course then makes her ask me why I didn't warn her how hard it can be to be pregnant. I didn't, because, for one thing, it's impossible to predict how anyone will feel during her pregnancy. Additionally, telling someone who really wants to conceive that pregnancy can pose challenges she hasn't even thought about doesn't seem like the best course of action. Besides, some women do feel fabulous for nine months (and for those of us who didn't, we can survive quite nicely without hearing how wonderful those women's pregnancies were, thank you very much!).

In subsequent chapters, I'm going to give you lots of advice on how to put all these conflicted feelings in perspective, how to cope with them, and how to lower their effect on you. But for now, let's take a look at the symptoms that commonly occur when you're expecting.

Frustrating Fatigue

Fatigue and pregnancy go hand in hand. In fact, fatigue is frequently the first pregnancy symptom that women notice. (The other common first is breast tenderness.) Pregnancy fatigue is unlike other kinds of fatigue; it makes you feel heavy and exhausted, not so much tired, but just burned out. It brings about a bone-deep weariness that has many women in bed, fast asleep, by 8:00 p.m.

Pregnancy fatigue seems insurmountable. Wake up from a two-hour nap, and rather than feeling refreshed, you want to roll over for another two hours. Sit down to read a book or watch television, and within seconds you're zonked out. Just the thought of lying down can make your eyelids heavy.

What causes this? The most likely culprits are the hormonal changes of pregnancy. Hormone levels boomerang during pregnancy, especially in the first few months. Another contributor is the fact that other pregnancy symptoms—for example, having to urinate more frequently—can interfere with your ability to get a good night's sleep. After all, it's hard to start the day feeling fabulous when you were up several times during the night to pee.

Stress and anxiety contribute to feelings of fatigue as well. Even low levels of stress or anxiety wear on you, increasing fatigue levels and making you feel less energetic. They also affect your ability to get the rest you need. Studies show that stress and anxiety have an effect on our ability to fall asleep, to stay asleep, and to wake up feeling refreshed. You need to remember that even positive things can make us feel stressed, and we all tend to feel stress when we are experiencing change. Some of the most stressful events in our lives are positive, such as getting married, buying a house, getting promoted, and of course having a baby. So even the happiest pregnant woman, if she is honest, might acknowledge some feelings of stress in the course of her nine months of expecting.

Fatigue can have an incredibly demoralizing effect on pregnant women—especially if you're young, healthy, and active. Many women have never felt this kind of fatigue before, unless they've had a bout of the flu. Active women I have worked with are shocked when they completely lose interest in their morning swim or their evening run, discovering that the climb up the stairs to bed at night is the only exercise they crave. And even when your doctor tells you that what you're feeling is normal, it's hard to imagine that it really is. It's also depressing to think that you'll be feeling so worn out for months and that you may have to give up your active lifestyle. One of my patients told me after her baby was born that she would have been better off taking her three-month maternity leave during the first trimester, when the brain fog of fatigue made her feel that she was completely ineffective at work. Too bad we can't all have two maternity leaves per baby.

The good news about pregnancy fatigue is that for most women it lets up during the second trimester (what I call the whirling dervish phase; you get your energy back, which is good because this is a great time to start getting ready for the baby), and although it can return during trimester three, it's usually not as bad as it was during those initial weeks. But as with most pregnancy symptoms, you can't always count on your body following the "typical" schedule. For some women, fatigue can last for a full forty weeks, while others find pregnancy brings with it a constant energy high.

Exhaustion would just descend on Carrie in the first trimester. She says, "I had extreme fatigue. I would hit a wall and need to sleep immediately. I didn't drive during that time, because I would be so overcome." Later in her pregnancy, Carrie would take naps when tired, but she wasn't hit with the same bone-crushing fatigue that got her in the first trimester.

Impish Insomnia

With all that fatigue, it might seem counterintuitive that most pregnant women experience insomnia. After all, when you are exhausted, sleep should come easily. Unfortunately, this isn't the case during pregnancy. Insomnia is one of the most frequently reported symptoms during pregnancy but also one of the least talked about. Getting up in the night to pee does not usually result in falling back to sleep immediately, because your mind tends to take over and you find yourself lying in bed, thinking and worrying and planning. Many of my patients find this so frustrating. They are exhausted and they crave sleep, but they lie in bed and worry that they aren't sleeping. There are many ways to learn how to sleep better during pregnancy, however, and we devote a chunk of chapter 5 to specific non-medication solutions. The main thing to focus on is to recognize that most pregnant women have problems getting a good night's sleep but there are ways to overcome your insomnia.

Anne was able to nap when she was tired, but when she was about seven months pregnant, she and her partner were in the process of buying a new home. This had her worrying about house issues as well as baby ones. "I would wake up at 3:00 a.m. and not be able to go back to sleep. I'd start thinking about questions and would Google them on my iPad. I'd go from link to link to link and get caught up in a whirlwind of things I probably didn't want to read about. I also couldn't get totally comfortable in bed. I had a wishbone pregnancy pillow (among others); my husband had a sliver of the bed, and the rest of it was pillows and me. Some days, I'd wake up early in the morning and just start *thinking*, then I'd fall back to sleep around 5:00 or 6:00. It's a good thing I could switch my work schedule to go in later, or I don't know how I would have managed with not being able to sleep and working."

Nasty Nausea

Next up on the pregnancy symptom hit parade is nausea. Personally, I refuse to refer to this noxious ordeal as "morning sickness" because I had it during both my pregnancies, and believe me, I *wish* it only transpired in the morning. Unfortunately, it can come on at any time of day (or all day). The low point of my second pregnancy? When my four-year-old realized that she could count the number of times I vomited. As in, "Guess what, Daddy? Mommy threw up *seven* times!"

Nausea occurs most often in early pregnancy, although for an unfortunate few it lingers longer. Typically, it disappears after the first trimester, when your body starts to get used to your hormone levels zigzagging all over the place. Some women have only occasional feelings of nausea. But others get extremely nauseated, with waves of discomfort accompanied by vomiting.

Even if you know that your pregnancy nausea is likely to disappear by thirteen weeks, you're still dealing with a lot of crummy feelings. I remember one day, early in my first pregnancy, hanging over the toilet with tears in my eyes, thinking, "I didn't sign up for this." Nobody wanted a baby more than I did, and yet, as I endured wave after wave of nausea, I questioned the whole idea of pregnancy—which left me feeling shocked, bewildered, and ashamed. If I couldn't handle a bit of nausea, I wondered, what kind of a mother would I be?

Arduous Anxiety

The definition of anxiety is a feeling of worry or nervousness, usually about the uncertain outcome of a future event. Anxiety occurs throughout life, but it is more likely to happen when we have something big on our radar screens for the near future—like, say, having a baby.

People are surprised when they hear about a pregnant woman's feeling anxious. What is there to be anxious about, they wonder, especially if you are having a healthy pregnancy? For one thing, worrying that you actually *are* having a healthy pregnancy—despite what your doctor says. Many women worry, and they worry because they care.

Pregnancy brings out our anxious inner voices the way few other life experiences do. I can't tell you how common it is for pregnant women to be plagued with anxiety. Here are just a few of the common questions that nag at them:

- Is my baby healthy?
- Am I healthy?
- What if something goes wrong with my baby or my pregnancy?
- Will I be able to endure labor and delivery?
- What if I do something embarrassing during labor?
- Will I be a good mother?
- Will my partner be a good parent?
- Will I ever lose all this weight I'm gaining?

- If I go back to work after my baby is born, will my baby get the right kind of care?
- If I follow my dream to be a stay-at-home mom, how will we pay our bills?
- Will I ever stop feeling so tired?
- Will I ever feel like myself again?

Isabella was very anxious during both of her pregnancies but for different reasons. She and her husband are carriers for a genetic disorder, so they needed to do genetic testing to make sure their babies were okay. She says the hardest thing about being pregnant was this: "Managing my anxiety. For the first, I had what I thought was 'normal' anxiety—is the baby okay, et cetera." Her first did not have the genetic disorder, but he was born premature. So, when she became pregnant a second time, she says, "I had a chest-crushing feeling; I was anxious about the testing, which was relieved when I got good results, but because I had previously given birth prematurely, I worried about what would be next. So, for the second pregnancy, I was anxious throughout the entire pregnancy. The reality of being pregnant is much more stressful than I could have imagined."

Bummed by the Blues

As I said earlier in the chapter, the symptoms of early pregnancy are a lot like the symptoms of depression. So sometimes it is hard to determine if you are feeling the normal sensations of a pregnant woman or if you are suffering from depression. Women who want to get pregnant might wonder why anyone lucky enough to conceive could possibly be depressed. But for many women, pregnancy poses a real challenge to their emotional well-being—especially if they have a history of depression. If you suspect that you are more depressed than run-of-the-mill hormonal, it is important to remember that any big life changes, even good ones, can trigger feelings of hopelessness and despair.

Because pregnancy mimics depression, to determine the cause of your symptoms you should focus on the emotional rather than the physical symptoms of depression. Ask yourself the following questions:

- Do I look forward to things the way I used to?
- Do I look forward to the future?
- Am I content or happy much of the time?
- Do I get as much pleasure from activities as I used to?
- Am I as interested in things as I used to be?

If you answered no to two or more questions, it is possible that you are in fact experiencing depression. But as you will read about later in this book, there are lots of ways to find relief from your symptoms and feel better during pregnancy.

Substantial Stress

Pregnancy has always caused stress, but it's even more stressful in today's overly wired world. When our moms were pregnant, they felt concerned about their pregnancy and their babies' health. But today, a pregnant woman's list of pressures is so much longer, fostered by social-media-fueled perfectionism, alarmist news reporting, celebrity baby-bump watching, and intense product marketing (of everything from natural baby care products and "green" nursery furniture to cord-blood-banking services and even Bellybuds, a specialized speaker system that pumps prenatal music and voices directly into a woman's bump during pregnancy). All of these contribute to a widespread belief that if you do everything just right, your baby—and your life—will be perfect.

Melissa, who became pregnant with a second child when her first was nineteen months old, felt stress and pressure. "I feel overwhelmed in not having enough time to do everything, but I tend to take on a lot. I wanted to decorate the nursery in a particular way, and being told no (that I couldn't paint while pregnant) or that I was taking on too much made me want to do it more. I have lots of plans. I know I have too much on my plate, but some of it is self-imposed. It's good to have things that I *want* to do. There are things I *should* do—like my husband's company party. But I like to use my time differently now."

The truth behind this stress-inducing perfectionism is

that you have much less control than you're being promised. In fact, many of the problems that occur in pregnancy are largely unpreventable. Not only that, but pregnancy tends to amplify any stresses that existed before conception, bumping up the stress in any situation—from problematic relationships and jobs to finances and health. The top three things that couples tend to fight about are money, sex, and kids—all issues that are central to becoming and being pregnant. Being pregnant can often be a catalyst for conflict, rather than the bonding experience that many couples anticipate. Many couples who decide to have a baby to improve or save their relationships find that the pregnancy only serves to drive them apart.

Although stress is a normal reaction to a new situation and there are multiple reasons why pregnant women feel stress and anxiety, it is important to find ways to reduce stress for your own peace of mind and the health of your baby. Research shows that excessive stress during pregnancy can be truly harmful: It's associated with premature birth and low birth weight, which can lead to a range of health problems for babies. In addition, having anxiety during pregnancy is a significant predictor of postpartum depression.

✧

You Don't Have to Experience
a Blissful Pregnancy to Be a Blissful Mother

Last week, I was talking to one of my colleagues, Gwenn, about this book. She laughed and told me a story about something that really surprised her during her second pregnancy. Gwenn had been pretty physically miserable during her first pregnancy—lots of nausea, some vomiting, and disabling fatigue for the first trimester. Apparently, her misery was visible to those around her, although she is now an extremely happy mother to her three-year-old son. Gwenn had a friend who had had two fantastic pregnancies—boundless energy, not a second of morning sickness—basically easy pregnancies from start to finish. When her friend heard that Gwenn was pregnant again and asked how she was feeling, Gwenn mentioned some early morning sickness. The friend responded, "Oh, that's right. I forgot that you hate being pregnant." Gwenn was shocked by this comment because although she didn't feel physically well while pregnant, emotionally she loved being pregnant. She hated the idea that she projected the image of being a miserable pregnant woman, when in fact she was thrilled to be pregnant with her second baby.

I have seen this same scenario so many times. Keep in mind that how you feel during pregnancy has no bearing on how you feel about becoming a mother. So although I have spent my entire career promoting the mind/body connection, I think pregnancy is an exception. I think it is entirely possible to feel lousy physically but still be happy about being pregnant.

Feeling Stressed?

Frankly, there are lots of things to be stressed-out about during pregnancy. And it is normal to feel stress to a certain degree. To get a sense of how stressed you are, and which aspects of pregnancy are wigging you out the most, take this quiz.

Quiz
How Stressed Are You About Being Pregnant?

1. How planned was this pregnancy?

a. *It happened right away.*
b. *It happened relatively quickly.*
c. *I had been trying for a long time.*
d. *It was totally unplanned.*

e. *I have no idea how I got pregnant unless it was another Immaculate Conception, or it is true that multiple margaritas cause pregnancy.*

2. How is your energy level?

a. *I have as much energy as I've ever had.*
b. *I usually feel pretty energetic, although sometimes I feel fatigued.*
c. *I do pretty well most of the time, but right now my eyelids are heavy, and I may not make it to the end of this quiz.*
d. *It's hard to find the energy to hold this book in my hand.*
e. *I feel so exhausted that I sometimes find myself going to bed before sunset.*

3. How often do you feel nauseated or need to vomit?

a. *I feel terrific; if I didn't know I was pregnant, I would never have guessed.*
b. *I feel pretty good most days, but I have to be careful about what I eat and I need to avoid certain smells.*
c. *My physical symptoms are really interfering with my quality of life.*
d. *I feel lousy most days; I am nauseated most of the time and vomit frequently.*

e. *I am so ticked off at my partner for knocking me up that I am tempted to give him syrup of ipecac so he knows what it feels like to vomit your guts up frequently.*

4. How are your anxiety levels?

a. *I feel normal, just the way I did before I got pregnant.*
b. *I usually feel okay, but sometimes I find myself worrying about the future.*
c. *I find myself worrying about my pregnancy with some regularity.*
d. *I worry so much that I'm getting worried about my worrying.*
e. *My anxiety is out of control; I watch others drink alcohol and have almost snatched their drinks out of their hands because I know I would feel less anxious with a good buzz.*

5. How stressed have you been feeling since you got pregnant?

a. *Not stressed at all. I feel blissful, just as I expected.*
b. *Most of the time I feel in control of my life, but I have occasional twinges of panic.*
c. *I am beginning to realize how much my life is going to change, and these feelings of panic hit me mostly at night.*

d. *I am a wreck. I am stressed about everything—the baby, my job, the house, our relationship; you name it, I am worried about it.*

e. *I am a complete stress machine. My obstetrician has offered me a sedative because I am bouncing off the walls.*

6. **How are the future grandparents doing?**

a. *They are beyond thrilled.*

b. *They are excited but unobtrusive.*

c. *They are mostly continuing to focus on their own lives.*

d. *They are calling every day and want to come to all my doctor's appointments.*

e. *If they show up in the delivery room, as they are threatening to do, I will throw the placenta at them.*

7. **How are you and your partner handling impending parenthood?**

a. *Wonderfully. He is so excited and wants to talk about the baby as much as I do.*

b. *Pretty well. He likes telling his friends about all the details.*

c. *So-so. He comes to the doctor's appointments when I ask but otherwise doesn't seem to be affected.*

d. *Not well. He doesn't seem interested and is worried he won't be able to watch as much sports on television once the baby comes.*

e. *He is in total denial that there is a baby coming and has asked for a paternity test.*

8. **How much do you worry about the pregnancy and the baby's health?**

a. *Not at all. I know that I am taking really good care of myself and the baby will be fine.*

b. *I think about it sometimes but am pretty confident that we will both be okay.*

c. *I call my obstetrician every week with questions and concerns.*

d. *I am really nervous about everything; I lie awake at night going over worst-case scenarios.*

e. *I am a complete wreck, and the more I worry, the more I know that there is something terribly wrong with the baby and it was caused by my worrying.*

9. **How depressed/sad are you feeling?**

a. *I feel happy all or most of the time.*

b. *I feel pretty normal, experiencing the ups and downs of daily life.*

c. *I have been feeling sad more often than happy and am worried that I am not happy enough about the baby coming.*

d. *I am really depressed but am embarrassed to tell people how much I am struggling. I either need to talk to someone or go on medication.*

e. *I am truly regretting throwing away my happy pills.*

10. Do you sometimes regret getting pregnant?

a. *Never.*

b. *Once in a while, I look forward to having pregnancy over with, but I'm usually okay with it.*

c. *I think about it a lot; it is beginning to scare me that this was a permanent decision.*

d. *I spend a lot of time second-guessing myself; this doesn't really feel like the best time to be having a baby.*

e. *I hate being pregnant, am convinced my baby will be ugly, and have covered all my mirrors so I don't need to see my horrible fat body.*

Scoring: Give yourself the following points for each answer you circled, then use the chart that follows to determine how stressed you are about being pregnant:

- Score 0 for each A answer.
- Score 1 for each B answer.
- Score 2 for each C answer.
- Score 3 for each D answer.
- Score 4 for each E answer.

Score	What It Means
0–7	You are remarkably calm and relaxed. You are (a) one of the luckiest women in the world or (b) in denial about your real feelings. Think about whether you're being honest with yourself.
8–15	You're on the cool side of normal; you've got some normal stresses, but overall you're in pretty good shape.
16–23	Like so many pregnant women, you feel stressed about some things and relaxed about others. Overall, though, you're right in the middle zone.
24–32	You've got a few stressors too many. Maybe your physical symptoms are extra annoying, or perhaps your worries are getting to you.
33–40	Being stressed during pregnancy is normal, but at this moment your stress levels are hitting the roof. Consider talking with your health-care provider about whether you have anxiety, depression, or other issues that need to be addressed professionally.

After you determine where you are on the stress scale, go back and look at the questions where you answered C, D, or E. Those are your major stress sources, and acknowledging them can be very helpful for you now and as you read the rest of the book. Pinpointing your stressors is the first step toward decreasing their effect on you. No matter where your score places you, this book can help you lower your stress levels, feel less anxious, and find more peace.

The Answer May Not Be in a Pill

Unfortunately, relief for all of the stress, anxiety, and moodiness of pregnancy doesn't come in a pill. Although 11 to 13 percent of pregnant women in the United States take antidepressant medications during at least part of their pregnancies, this is not a good choice for many pregnant women. As one of my psychiatrist colleagues said to me last week, no psychiatrist wants to put a pregnant woman on medication unless he or she has to.

Several colleagues and I were interested in understanding how antidepressants affect mothers and babies. We were particularly intrigued by the effects of selective serotonin reuptake inhibitors, or SSRIs, which are the most commonly prescribed antidepressants (they include Celexa, Lexapro, Paxil, Prozac, and Zoloft). So we conducted a review of published studies that evaluated the outcomes for women who took SSRI antidepressants during pregnancy. The results of our analysis, which were published in 2013 in the journal *Human Reproduction*, startled us.

We found that taking SSRIs during pregnancy can increase the risk of a range of complications, including the following:

- miscarriage
- congenital abnormalities (such as heart defects)

- preterm birth (birth before thirty-seven weeks)
- neonatal health complications, such as low birth weight and respiratory distress
- newborn behavioral syndrome, which is associated with persistent crying, jitteriness, difficulty feeding, and in rare cases seizures and breathing difficulties requiring intubation
- delayed motor development in babies and toddlers
- autism (a twofold increased risk of autism spectrum disorders)

∽

Dos and Don'ts If You Are Taking an SSRI

- **Don't** stop taking your medication without speaking to your health-care provider.
- **Do** learn about alternatives to medication to treat depressive symptoms.
- **Don't** panic. The vast majority of babies whose moms took SSRIs during pregnancy are fine.
- **Do** review your own history with successful use of other therapies, such as cognitive behavioral therapy and exercise.
- **Don't** make any decision in a panic. Take your time.
- **Do** think carefully about the risk-benefit ratio for you when you make the decision.

Although there are risks, should SSRIs ever be prescribed during pregnancy? The answer is yes. In the case of serious depression, it can make sense for doctors to prescribe them—provided they do so cautiously and the woman and her partner receive counseling about the potential risks as well as the benefits. There are many women who truly need to take medication for their depression during their pregnancy. Depressive symptoms during pregnancy should not go untreated, but antidepressants are not the only treatment available. You'll be glad to know there is a lot you can do for yourself during pregnancy to ease your physical and psychological symptoms.

One of the best non-pharmacological treatments for depression is cognitive behavioral therapy (CBT), a type of psychotherapy that focuses on the connections between thoughts, feelings, and behaviors. All of the mind/body treatments that I teach in this book, in my practice, and at the Domar Center are built on the principles of CBT. (See appendix I for mind/body techniques you can use in your pregnancy and beyond.)

Other non-pharmaceutical options that can successfully reduce depression in pregnant women without putting their babies at risk include other forms of psychotherapy, exercise, yoga, acupuncture, massage, and nutritional supplements— all of which I'll tell you more about later in this book.

Pregnancy can be amazing and anxiety producing— frequently at the same time. The good news (in addition to your being pregnant) is that you *can* cope with what is driving you crazy, whether it is your hormones or your mother-in-law. When you better understand the internal and external forces that are causing you to feel the way you do, when you realize that you are not the only one to feel this way about (or during) pregnancy, when you learn that there are lots of ways to ease your symptoms and ride out the rough patches, you can find peace of mind (and body) during your pregnancy.

Chapter 2

Pregnancy Perfection

THE MEDIA AREN'T very good for pregnant women. How many pregnant women do you know (including yourself) who feel better about themselves after looking at any magazine photo spread on pregnancy? Seriously, have you ever seen pictures of stretch marks? From Facebook to Internet pregnancy sites, from product marketing to online medical columns, from mommy bloggers to celebrity "bump-watch" Web sites, women face a nonstop barrage of unrealistic expectations about what they should do, feel, look like, weigh, think, eat, and buy while they are pregnant. It is relentless, and to protect themselves, women need to be aware of the effect that this flood of information and images from the media can have on anxiety and stress levels. At least once a week, I tell a patient to stop looking at the

Internet, because doing so is making her so miserable and feel as if she has lost control of her body.

On the Magazine Stands, on the Web

"Kate's Baby Joy! A Playmate for George—But Another Tough Pregnancy" (People magazine)—on Duchess Kate's morning sickness

"Mila Delivery Room Drama!" (OK! magazine)—on Mila Kunis's delivery

"Portia's Already Gained 10 lbs" (Star magazine)—on Portia de Rossi's pregnancy, which later turned out to be a false report

"Eva Mendes Flaunts Slim Post-Baby Bod Just 4 Months After Birth of Baby" (hollywoodlife.com)—slim celebrity report

"See Zoe Saldana's Amazing Post Baby Physique on the Oscars Red Carpet" (instyle.com)—it went on to say, "Can you believe Zoe Saldana gave birth to twin boys less than two months ago?"

Frankly, it is normal to feel anxious when you don't have control, and there is no time in your life when you have less control over your body and your emotions than when you are pregnant. Many pregnant women feel very vulnerable (and under the social microscope). They are surrounded by so many people who are constantly giving advice (most unsolicited) that is often not only contradictory but downright wrong. In the old days, women probably went to Mom or Grandma for advice, but now the World Wide Web and every stranger on the street are a source of information, advice, and stories. In addition, pregnant women are a perfect target for advertising and marketers because they are on the cusp of making big-ticket purchases and at a time when they very much want to do things right. This creates a perfect storm for merchandisers to tap into pregnant women's vulnerabilities while going for their wallets.

While not having control isn't appealing and can feel uncomfortable, remember that pregnancy isn't forever and that the result will be *your* baby. As a matter of fact, not having full control of your life during pregnancy is actually good training for when your baby arrives. I am always telling my patients that pregnancy seems to be designed to prepare you for motherhood. Sleep deprivation during pregnancy can make you adapt to functioning on less sleep, which comes in awfully handy during the newborn period. Having your pregnant body change prepares you for breast-feeding, and cravings and nausea may prepare you for having so little time to prepare food for yourself that you spend a couple of years surviving on leftover mac and cheese and the crusts from PB&Js.

Pregnancy Unveiled

In the past, pregnant women were hidden from the world. Literally. Women didn't appear in public once they started showing. In the last thirty-five years, so much has changed. Princess Diana caused shock by wearing a bikini when she was pregnant and showing ("Itsy-bitsy suit for mum-to-be," said England's *Daily Star* in 1981). Demi Moore's cover of *Vanity Fair* (1991) featuring her naked and pregnant was a first. Since then, many stars and performers have appeared on magazine covers and in other media naked and pregnant. Today, pregnancy is out there, and you can't miss baby bumps both covered and uncovered. People talk, think, and behave differently about pregnancy than in the past.

While it's great that pregnancy is viewed as something that doesn't need to be hidden from the world anymore, there are some problems with the way the media cover pregnancy. First, they are not photographing or celebrating the pregnancy of the average woman. They are featuring stories about women who are actors, models, or performers and whose livelihoods depend on being in excellent photogenic shape—no matter what. They had fabulous figures and were incredibly fit going into their pregnancies (thanks to personal chefs, fitness trainers, and so on), and don't forget the magic of Photoshop. So comparing yourself with any of these women is an exercise in automatically feeling badly about how you look while pregnant. Additionally, the media never talk about how it is normal for a woman to get round when she is pregnant. Either they are touting how thin she looks (thin equals good in media-speak), or they are bewailing how much weight she's put on. Usually this is phrased as "So-and-so is really packing on the pounds!" It gets worse when they run the "body after baby" features, which seem intended to shame the women who don't immediately drop all their baby weight and skip out of the hospital in their skinny jeans.

Here's something to think about next time you see one of those annoying "Body After Baby" or "Bye-Bye, Baby Weight" articles. I recently met with several therapists who work with infertility patients across the country including actresses, models, and musicians. A little-known fact is that quite a number of celebrities are now using gestational surrogates to carry their pregnancies and are wearing pregnancy pillows to appear as if they were carrying their child-to-be. So before you make yourself crazy with envy over the flat-within-six-weeks belly, look for her pregnancy pictures. If her face looks the same throughout her "pregnancy," it is very possible that she was never pregnant in the first place!

Seeing those features sets up women to worry (largely unnecessarily) about how much weight they are gaining during their real-life pregnancy and how hard it might be to lose it after the baby is born. I can't tell you how many of my patients were miserable after seeing photographs of Duchess Kate's totally flat stomach, mere weeks after the births of Prince George and Princess Charlotte.

Another negative offshoot of the media's feeling free to comment on all aspects of pregnancy is that it seems to grant license for anyone, and I mean anyone, to comment about you and your bump. Women seem to become community property when they are pregnant. You might have experienced this yourself. Have you had a co-worker touch your belly without asking? I have a friend who is a lawyer, and when she was about eight months pregnant with her first child, she was in court, and the opposing lawyer reached out and touched her belly, during a trial! Do strangers in elevators opine about the sex of your baby? Have people ever said to you, "I hope you are doing _____," or "You're not going to eat that, are you?" Has their uninvited "advice" caused you to panic and worry that you've done something to permanently damage your child? The media and the self-appointed "pregnancy police" can make you feel as though you are being assaulted with what to do and what not to do, making you feel as though you are not measuring up to some ideal standard.

The media aren't all bad. On the plus side, they have helped to normalize pregnancy, but I really wish they would be more forgiving about women as they gain weight—which is a normal result of pregnancy. Another benefit of what seems like obsessive celebrity-baby-bump-watch media is that occasionally a woman in the media will have a common pregnancy-related issue and the coverage not only gets the issue into the spotlight but also helps women feel that they are not the only ones. For example, Kate Middleton (the Duchess of Cambridge) has experienced horrible morning sickness during both of her pregnancies and required hospitalization. Having an issue like acute morning sickness out in the open can help women if they are dealing with that issue themselves. In general, however, the media portray the "ideal" rather than the "real." The reality is more often vomiting and hemorrhoids, not spending forty weeks 24/7 blissfully awaiting the arrival of the perfect baby.

Quiz
Perfectly Pregnant?

⸙

1. How much time, on average, do you spend online on pregnancy-related matters?

   a. *Less than half an hour per day.*
   b. *Half an hour to two hours per day.*
   c. *Two to four hours per day.*

d. *I'm checking constantly. I have every pregnancy-related app on the market and dozens of bookmarked Web sites.*

2. **How vigilant are you about celebrity pregnancies?**

a. *A Kardashian is pregnant?*
b. *I only keep track of who is married versus not married when pregnant. I glance at the magazines at the grocery store checkout counter to see who's expecting.*
c. *I'm the first in my office to know that a celeb baby is on the way.*
d. *I know the due date and gender of every famous bump-to-be.*

3. **How much do you follow the advice you read on Web sites?**

a. *I have my doctor on speed dial and always go to her before the Internet.*
b. *I read a few sponsored and government Web sites, and if I can't find corroborated information, I ask my doctor.*
c. *If I read an alarming thing, I stop and talk to my partner about it or bring it up to my doctor.*
d. *I program just about any advice I get from the Internet into my phone and follow it to a T. I eat kale at every meal and drink gallons of water because I read online that it will raise my baby's IQ.*

4. **What do you do if your favorite Web site and your OB disagree?**

a. *I go with my OB unless there are two doctors in the practice and they disagree. In that case, I might go to the Web to act as a mediator.*

b. *I'll go with my OB unless he or she isn't as current as the Web site.*

c. *I give equal weight to the Web and my OB. I go with whatever matches my gut feeling.*

d. *I tend to believe what I read online. Ten thousand women are on the Web site, and he only sees a few hundred. There is safety in numbers.*

5. **How much do celebrity pregnancies influence yours?**

a. *I don't pay attention to celebrity bumps. Half the time, magazines say someone is pregnant when she's really just wearing a baggy shirt.*

b. *I am most interested in celebrities who are due at the same time as I am, so I can compare bumps.*

c. *I check on Web sites and see if I want to look at products a celebrity recommends.*

d. *I follow them on Twitter and, when I can afford it, buy exactly what a celebrity wears, eat what she eats, and shop where she shops.*

Scoring: Give yourself the following points for each answer you circled, then use the chart that follows to determine how stressed you are about being pregnant:

- Score 0 for each A answer.
- Score 1 for each B answer.
- Score 2 for each C answer.
- Score 3 for each D answer.

Score	What It Means
0–3	You are one mellow pregnant gal. Keep up the good work.
4–7	You still fall into the normal range; nice.
8–11	You need to shift your attention inward and learn to trust your gut feeling more. Your body, your baby.
12–15	There is such a thing as being too perfect. You need to challenge some of your internal chatter and let more slide off your back. Keep on reading the next few chapters for suggestions.

Pregnancy Pressure

A big result of all this celebrity pregnancy media is that it creates a set of false standards that you may feel you have to follow in order to have a great pregnancy. You are supposed to look fabulous, radiant, glowing, and essentially like your old self with a barely noticeable bump. But the reality is that your body changes during pregnancy. Your breasts get larger, your hips can expand, and you may gain weight in your face, thighs, or arms. *And it's normal!* Repeat after me: "Normal!" But these fake expectations also spill over into how you "should" feel during pregnancy. There is no room for any negativity because you must be happy, grateful, appreciative, vibrant, and optimistic. Let's face it; most of us are not all of these things in our daily lives, let alone when we are facing a transformative event that affects us physically and emotionally.

Things also get a little crazy when it comes to eating while pregnant. Pregnant women often overemphasize the effect of their nutrition on the baby. And they can make themselves anxious and stressed when they attempt to eat and live perfectly. Yes, avoiding alcohol, cigarettes, and drugs is a must, but other than that, simply eating good food is the best approach to maintaining your health along with your baby's. Your baby's nutritional needs are actually relatively modest. Media, blogs, and chat rooms on Web sites can make it seem as if what you eat will determine your kid's SAT score and future life success, which inspires or guilts many women into scrutinizing every morsel they eat. They fear that if they don't eat perfectly nutritiously, they can compromise their health or the development of the baby. I was incredibly nauseated during both of my pregnancies, and for some reason during my first pregnancy the only food that appealed to me was chocolate chip muffins from Dunkin' Donuts. I used to joke that my older daughter is constituted of those muffins and Tums. But I also worried a lot about the effect this limited diet would have on her development. The worrying was for naught. She met all her developmental milestones and is now in college. And, surprisingly enough, shows less fondness for chocolate chip muffins than her little sister!

On the other hand, there's the pregnancy myth that being pregnant gives you "permission" to eat whatever you want—that old wives' tale of "eating for two." Unfortunately, that is not the case. The problem is that many women, prior to becoming pregnant, have devoted a lot of time and energy restricting their eating and controlling their weight through diet and/or exercise. They just can't do the same thing during pregnancy, and it can throw them for a loop. Either they totally indulge: I had a patient who thought it was okay to eat bowls of mashed potatoes with a heaping bowl of ice cream for dessert—at every meal. That's not okay, because she ended up gaining far too much weight during her pregnancy and then struggled to take it off after the baby was born. Or, some women continue to try to restrict their eating, which can be bad for the baby's growth. Neither extreme is good. The best approach is to eat a bit more than you would normally eat but reduce fish and avoid listeria-prone foods like unpasteurized milk and dairy products or cold cuts and hot dogs. When in doubt about what to eat or how much, ask your OB. You will be weighed at each visit, so both of you will have a good sense of whether or not you are gaining weight at an appropriate pace. But all of this focus on how you "should" look, feel, and eat can contribute to your feeling stressed, inadequate, and unattractive.

Many of my patients bemoan the fact that they have a Facebook friend or someone they know on Instagram who posts photographs of her pregnant self looking fantastic and bragging about her minimal weight gain and how fabulously her pregnancy is going. You have to remember that a lot of women cop the Mommy Superior attitude because they want to make themselves feel better. So, while she may be posting a flat-stomached photograph of herself in a bikini at sixteen weeks, what she is not posting is how many times she threw up that morning or how she is feeling depressed, despite how she looks. Social media invite us to put our best face forward. Consumers of social media can feel as if they don't measure up. Researchers at the University of Missouri have found that Facebook can lead to symptoms of depression if the site triggers feelings of envy among its users.[1]

A few years ago, one of my patients asked me if it was healthy to compare oneself with others. Good question. I responded that in fact research shows that when we compare ourselves with people less fortunate, comparing down, we get psychologically healthier. But in fact, what do we tend to do? We compare up. When I drive my ten-year-old minivan with more than 100,000 miles on it, I am not comparing it with the rusted wreck behind me held together with duct tape. Instead, I am focusing on the sporty BMW that just cut me off. Yes, I know that the BMW won't haul half my younger daughter's soccer team or everything my older daughter needed to take to college, but it's human nature to be drawn to what is "better" than what we have. We seek up.

We all tend to compare up, and seeing someone who appears to be having an effortless pregnancy can contribute to your feeling as if you were doing something wrong. Chances are, you are doing just fine! Also remember all your pregnant friends and acquaintances who are far rounder, pimpled, and stretch marked than you who would never post anything online. Only the perfect post.

Brittany, thirty-seven, thought she would be glowing and happy during her pregnancy. She discovered that what she thought and the reality were like night and day. She was nauseated most of the time and had to seek treatment for back pain caused by pressure from the baby. She had some friends who were pregnant at the same time, but instead of bonding with them, she said she felt like "the odd duck out." She explains, "My friend having her first said she was so happy that she could be pregnant all the time. My other friend who was having her second only complained about being hot. I was jealous because I was sick day and night and had a lot of back pain."

Social media can actually be helpful and supportive in some circumstances. There are pregnancy boards and Web sites that may help you feel less isolated; you can share your hopes and fears in a supportive environment, be part of a tribe, and communicate with others who know what you are going through. It feels terrific to have someone else post exactly what you are thinking or feeling but may be too embarrassed to discuss with a family member or friend. Many of my patients tell me that one of the best things about seeing me is that it is the only safe place where they can complain about their pregnancy. These boards can serve the same purpose. You can vent, bitch, and complain to your heart's content and not worry that you will offend anyone or lead anyone in your life to believe that you don't want to be pregnant. And, frankly, just because you complain about being pregnant or how you feel while you are pregnant doesn't mean you don't want to be pregnant or have a baby.

Please remember that if you spend every waking moment of the forty weeks agonizing over every bite you take and every ounce you gain, you will miss something very profound: You are making a baby! The truth is that a baby takes over the body, and it is supposed to. You may break out, gain weight in places you don't expect (face, thighs, arms), and be puffy and swollen so that your rings and shoes feel tight. Nothing of this is out of the ordinary. It is simply what often happens to a pregnant body. And, remember, it's temporary. Which is one of the best things about pregnancy. There is an end date. And on that end date your baby is born!

Layettes, Strollers, and Onesies, Oh My!

Another area where women feel enormous pressure is in filling up the nursery with the latest, best, most safe, educationally sound, and IQ-enhancing gadgets, furniture, and transportation devices. There is pressure to register for tons of stuff, most of which you can probably do without or borrow. Ask other moms what has worked for them. They can tell you what you really need. Make a list of must-haves versus want-to-haves.

Magazines feature lists and checklists for outfitting your baby that are largely driven not by you and your baby's best interests but by the magazines' wanting to keep advertisers happy. You will see features in magazines of celebrity nurseries or "which stroller did this star buy," and in most cases the strollers, cribs, and so on are all top-of-the-line, high-end equipment—in other words, the most expensive version of stroller imaginable. It's hard to resist reading these features and articles. You will be drawn to all things pregnancy in a way you might not ever have thought possible. It's all part of the phenomenon that I call "preg-dar," where a pregnant woman is immediately drawn to any and all news or information about pregnancy, birth, and babies. This means that you will see pregnant women everywhere you go and notice more baby items than you ever noticed before; your antennae will be tuned to every feature on the news or Web about recalls for things like strollers and cribs. Hearing about these risks can raise your anxiety levels and make you scared to purchase one product or another.

You may also feel pressured to spend as much as possible to ensure that you get "the best." If you and your partner are already having tense discussions over finances, all of this spending can add stress to your relationship, not to mention your budget. Hopefully, you will not be the only ones shopping for your baby; often family members offer to pitch in with outfitting the baby and purchasing furniture and other items. But while it can be great if your parents offer to outfit the nursery, if your partner's parents offer to do the same, you will be caught in the middle. Sometimes there is an economic difference between the in-laws, and one side can afford more extravagant gifts than the other, which can lead to resentment, grumbling, and you caught in the middle (again!).

The pressure to have a baby-stuff shopping spree is largely fueled by advertisers and marketers, but there is something else going on too. Many women feel that if they don't buy every possible item, everything that is "the best," and get everything brand-new, they are somehow doing a disservice to their baby. Even buying the bare necessities can cost a lot; if you insist on purchasing only top-of-the-line merchandise, you are going to be spending a great deal of money on things you probably don't need (and possibly can't afford). I recommend resisting the temptation to buy everything new. It's hard, but hand-me-downs (especially for newborns) are a great way to go. Those tiny clothes don't get worn for long, because babies can grow so fast. Ask around—a friend, a sibling, or a co-worker may have baby items that he or she no longer needs and would be happy to hand on to you. It can definitely be worth it. I had a patient who bought all new, expensive infant clothes, and she bought a lot. She didn't count on her baby's growing so fast. A brand-new outfit that she put on her son one morning was too small at the end of the day. Literally. When in doubt, buy a size up. You may need a few newborn-sized items, but the baby will grow and the clothes won't.

So how do you resist and keep yourself and your credit card from going into overdrive? You need to be aware of a couple of things:

- What you see in magazines is "aspirational" as determined by the media.
- What you see is an attempt to get you to buy something.
- They want to tap into your fear or guilt or desire to have and be the best.

- They want you to buy, and they want you to buy in quantity.
- The pregnant women you see in magazines and on TV are not real (and they have probably not paid retail for the items they are wearing or using). They've been Photoshopped, they are genetically gifted, and they have personal trainers and chefs to keep them looking great. As my friend Loretta LaRoche says, they pay someone to lift their legs.

What you see on social media may also be distorted. Although we all know someone who uses social media posts as an opportunity to catalog her agonies, most people tend to paint themselves in the best light possible. People post wonderful, happy vacation photographs but not photographs of doing laundry when they get home. People stretch the truth all the time. Be suspicious: The more someone trumpets how great things are, the more she may be overcompensating for her own worries and concerns. The more triumphant the post, the more suspicious I would get.

Pregnancy Web

Pregnant women are quick to hop on the Web to look for information, even before they have had their first visit with their OB. According to researchers at Penn State, "We found that first-time moms were upset that their first prenatal visit did not occur until eight weeks into pregnancy," said Jennifer L. Kraschnewski, assistant professor of medicine and public health sciences at the Penn State College of Medicine. "These women reported using Google and other search engines because they had a lot of questions at the beginning of pregnancy, before their first doctor's appointment." She pointed out that the regulation of medical information on the Internet is rare, which could be problematic and lead to alarming patients unnecessarily.[2]

The average woman spends approximately four hours a day on the Internet. There are a zillion pregnancy Web sites, and research has shown that over half the medical information on Internet sites is wrong. *Beware* and be very careful about taking the information on a site at face value—especially if the information is increasing your stress or anxiety. Confirm the facts with your doctor or nurse-midwife before getting upset or taking action. The best idea is to seek out information on government sites like the Centers for Disease Control (CDC) and well-established organizations like the American Heart Association, the American Academy of Pediatrics, and the American College of Obstetricians and Gynecologists. If you read something that bothers you, please try to confirm the accuracy on an official site of an organization that provides information or care to pregnant women. But always remember that your own healthcare provider knows you and your body better than any

Web site, blog, or chat room. If it is a pressing issue, call your doctor. If it seems like something that can wait, make a note of it in your smart phone or on a piece of paper and bring it up at your next appointment.

You also need to remember that most commercial sites are just that, commercial. They are trying to sell you something. As a pregnant woman who is going to be a big consumer of multiple products first during your pregnancy and then for your baby, you are a huge target for many companies. There is a feeding frenzy of shopping that you are invited to join, but before you jump in, be sure that you are making an informed choice and not being unduly influenced by marketing and ads.

When it comes to blogs and chat rooms, the same caveat applies. Most chat rooms and blogs are not moderated by experts, and posts are not vetted. While they can be a source of solace, the information may tend more toward opinions than facts. On many sites, you will find extremes— the absolute worst-case scenario or completely problem-free pregnancies. The reality lies somewhere in the middle. Look to the source; for example, chats/blogs on WebMD are relatively well vetted. But many other chat rooms and blogs (and sometimes the media) can spread misinformation like wildfire.

Here is an example: I was looking at the patient section of the Web site of a well-known infertility company. A headline proclaimed that brussels sprouts increased fertility. This intrigued me, because I didn't know of any study that showed that any food could increase fertility. So I investigated the story and discovered the source of that "fact." An article had appeared in a British newspaper noting that births in the U.K. peaked nine months after the month when brussels sprouts sales were at their highest. Its conclusion was that clearly brussels sprouts led to fertility. Ridiculous. There were likely a million other things that happened nine months earlier, only one of which involved the sale of brussels sprouts. But I can very well imagine desperate infertility patients reading that article, dutifully eating brussels sprouts by the pound, and futilely waiting for them to work their magic.

For the most part, information from much of the media is factual, but it doesn't replace speaking with a doctor or a nurse-midwife. Remember, the media are looking to promote stories that are newsworthy and have attention-getting information. They talk about the really bad or the really good. They often go for the shocking or the abnormal. In all likelihood, your pregnancy is neither shocking nor abnormal, but there may be a lot of influences on you that can make you feel as if it were.

There Is an App for That

Some women enjoy using smart-phone apps that will feed them daily or weekly information on the development of their baby. Apps can be fun, but all caveats on knowing the source of the information apply, and don't be surprised or concerned if your symptoms or size don't match up exactly with what pops up on your smart phone. As always, if you have concerns, raise them with your OB or nurse-midwife.

At twenty-four weeks, Holly really enjoys using an app. "Apps have been very helpful for me to keep track of development. It makes me feel more connected to her to see how she is developing. My husband is enjoying the updates. He'll ask, 'What size fruit is she today?'" Holly says. "I also go online and look up specific issues—like is it okay to fly when you are pregnant." As much as she appreciates the technology, however, she notes that "the Internet is convenient and can be a blessing but sometimes it's bad because you can diagnose yourself with anything! You can drive yourself crazy—the more you read, the more you know, but I'm trying to err on the side of less is better."

Why You Feel the Way You Do

The first time you are pregnant, everything is new and potentially weird, and every pregnant woman needs constant reassurance that what she is experiencing is normal. Sadly, the media aren't going to provide that. Normal doesn't sell. And, sadly, we can't always trust our friends to tell the truth either. They may hold back to spare our feelings (and worry), they may sanitize their experience to make themselves look good or to feel better, and, unfortunately, women can be competitive over something like pregnancy. They can feel resentful if you have an easy pregnancy and they didn't or get competitive over weight gain (and subsequent loss). Also, we all have that friend who is happy to share all the gory details of her pregnancy whether you want to hear them or not. Then there are the people who gleefully share the horrifying story of a friend of a friend of a friend that they swear is true. Why people feel the need to repeat these stories is a total mystery to me.

To reduce your anxiety about anything you read, hear, or see, as mentioned above, you can take it all with a grain of salt. Then check the information out with a trusted resource like your doctor or nurse-midwife.

⚲

Checking It Out

- Know your source. The best data come from studies that are randomized, controlled trials, published in a medical journal that has been peer-reviewed. Know that the bigger the publication (such as *Obstetrics and Gynecology*), the more scrutiny the information or study has gone under. Also check out any financial relationships the authors might have with the product.

- Go to reputable Web sites (that is, those ending in .gov or .org).
- Don't take your friend's word for it; double-check with your doctor or medical professional.
- Don't fall for the over-sharing syndrome in social media; usually the best and the worst of any situation are portrayed there. The middle ground and the most common experiences are rarely posted.

The media can be relentless. The aspirational portrayal of the perfect woman and the push to sell products don't stop when you are pregnant. In fact, they can feel more intense because the stakes seem higher now that you are going to become a mom. Because it's unrealistic to go on a media blackout for nine months, you need to approach what you see with a fresh and wary perspective. Armed with the knowledge that most women don't go through pregnancy as celebrities do, remember that commercial sites are trying to sell you something. Knowing that much of what you are experiencing is normal should help you to take the anxiety down a notch. But always resist the urge to compare yourself with friends or the fabulous photo spread in your favorite magazine.

Chapter 3

Pregnancy Survival Kit

PREGNANCY IS AN exciting time spent planning for the birth of your child and the positive changes that a new baby will bring to your life. Something I encourage my patients to work on during pregnancy is cultivating resilience. Resilience will help you to cope with any stresses that come your way during your nine months of pregnancy and beyond. In the same way that you might prepare a bag or a suitcase that will come to the hospital with you when you are ready to deliver, I encourage you to collect coping mechanisms to deal with any issues that come up during your pregnancy.

Pregnancy, as I'm sure you have discovered, can be all encompassing. It can affect your mental and physical health, your relationships, your finances, and your job/career—truly any and all aspects of your life. It's an exciting game changer, but, strangely enough, I do believe that the uncertainty, the lack of sleep, and, yes, the worry all prepare you for when you will have a new baby in your life.

Because feeling stressed and anxious can be a normal reaction during pregnancy, it's important to learn skills that will help you to reduce your worries so that you don't get caught up in a loop of blame or shame about anything to do with your pregnancy. These tools will come in handy now as well as later, when you are facing any challenging situation. You will be able to say to yourself, "I've got this!" rather than feeling as if you were stuck or overwhelmed. Like many psychologists, I believe that for the vast majority of my patients the answer to coping with stress, anxiety, and depression lies not in medication but in developing a range of effective skills that are described in this chapter.

Many Pregnant Women Cope by . . .

Complaining. They complain to their partner, mom, or friends. They go online to find blogs and chat rooms where (on the plus side) they realize they are not alone but (on the minus side) they are exposed to a host of pregnancy "truths" that just aren't true. Other women suffer in silence. Many don't feel comfortable complaining. They can also feel guilty for complaining about something that is supposed to be wonderful (especially if they have been through infertility treatments or taken a long time to get pregnant). If a pregnancy is a happy accident or otherwise unexpected, then it is easier to admit to suffering. But if a woman has carefully planned or worked to get pregnant, it feels ungrateful to be anything other than happy and uncomplaining.

Liz and her husband sought help for their infertility issue. She said, "We had one IVF with a miscarriage, and that was not easy for either of us." But they got through it and tried again. Now she is happily pregnant but a little conflicted. They did not let people know they had done IVF to get pregnant. "People didn't really know how lucky we felt." At the same time, when she was experiencing heartburn and hemorrhoids, she felt she couldn't really talk about her uncomfortable physical symptoms. "After all the effort we went through to get pregnant, I want to complain but feel guilty about it. I asked to be pregnant. I wanted this."

To be constantly overjoyed and without complaint through the nine months of pregnancy is unrealistic. However, there is plenty you can do to feel better when physical or emotional discomfort strikes.

Quiz
How Do You Cope?

1. **What is your history of taking medication to treat anxiety and/or depression?**

   a. *I have never taken medication.*
   b. *I have taken meds in the past, but not for a while.*
   c. *I was taking meds prior to this pregnancy but stopped before conceiving.*
   d. *I currently take several antidepressant and antianxiety meds during this pregnancy.*

2. **How do you cope when stressed?**

   a. *I have a therapist who has helped me in the past, and I touch base when I'm feeling anxious, stressed, or depressed.*
   b. *I've taken yoga, practiced meditation—you name it, I've tried it.*
   c. *I've been in therapy off and on.*
   d. *I currently take several antidepressant and antianxiety meds during this pregnancy.*

3. **How do you act when you are stressed?**

   a. *I keep a list of the things that help me feel better when wigging out—like take a walk or meditate.*
   b. *I talk to my partner or a friend.*
   c. *I distract myself by watching TV.*
   d. *I head for the fridge or freezer for comfort foods.*

4. **What does your negative self-talk sound like?**

   a. *I don't let it rule my thoughts. It's tough, but if I'm diligent, it works.*
   b. *It comes and goes. I've learned to distract myself.*
   c. *Sounds just like my mother.*
   d. *It is omnipresent. I know I am my own worst enemy, but I can't help myself.*

5. **Are you aware of your mood swings?**

   a. *I know that pregnant women can be volatile, so I'm learning to accept my mood swings (even if my partner isn't), and I'm working on finding ways to pamper myself and de-stress.*
   b. *I'm beginning to identify the triggers that make me go off the deep end.*
   c. *I'm very aware of my mood swings, but at least I recognize when I'm off the rails.*
   d. *I find myself feeling anxious and upset most of the time.*

6. What is your experience with mind/body skills?

a. *I've tried several, and they have helped in the past; I need to remind myself to use them.*

b. *I have done yoga and my partner runs, but I've never done any woo-woo stuff.*

c. *I've tried it in the past; nothing clicked for me.*

d. *None, I just live life.*

Scoring: Give yourself the following points for each answer you circled, then use the chart that follows to determine how stressed you are about being pregnant:

- Score 0 for each A answer.
- Score 1 for each B answer.
- Score 2 for each C answer.
- Score 3 for each D answer.

Score	What It Means
0–4	You are a pro at self-care! You have learned what you need—either that, or this is your sixth pregnancy and experience counts.
5–9	You are in a good place most of the time. It's likely you worry more about going off the deep end than you need to. Pat yourself on the back more.
10–14	This book is really good timing for you. It's as if you know what you need but you haven't figured out how to get there.

Score	What It Means
15–18	Whoa! Slow down, take a deep breath, and think about what you need and what you can get from those around you. The timing is good; you need to learn to care for yourself more effectively before you can take on another responsibility. Read on!

A Better Way to Cope

Although pregnancy may seem to create very different worries and anxieties from other life events, you have undoubtedly dealt with some conflict or issue in your past and been able to handle it. Draw on those inner resources now. Have you lost a grandparent, dealt with a parent's illness, helped a friend with a tragedy or loss, or seen some unhappiness or conflict in your life? Have you suffered from depression or anxiety?

Trust me, you have come out of those experiences with more wisdom than you may realize. Think carefully about times in the past when you had to cope with a challenge, and remember what worked to help you feel better. Also think about things you tried that didn't do you all that much good. So, for example, if something worked for you when your grandma died, it might work for you when dealing with the challenges of pregnancy. Maybe you had a long talk with your sister about how you miss your grandmother, and it made you feel better. Or you learned that the best way to deal with your boss's mood swings was to take long walks at lunchtime. When you got dumped by a boyfriend in high school, what worked and what didn't? It's very helpful to draw on your life experience to see what helped and what didn't so that you can use those skills now.

Perhaps a co-worker or friend is also pregnant (ideally within a few weeks of you), and you can speak to her. She may be grappling with the same issue as you are and can share some helpful coping ideas or a new perspective. Joan struggled with infertility and has a seven-and-a-half-year-old and, after years of trying, an eight-month-old. She has this advice: "Talk to someone who has a positive influence on you. It's hard to deal with all of this on your own, especially if you are having difficulties." Joan found it helpful to talk to her spouse, her mother, and her therapist.

Cultivating Resilience

To maintain your emotional health during pregnancy, you need to draw on your resilience or develop new skills. We all have coping mechanisms that we use when faced with challenges and demands. Some are healthier than others; mindful meditation rather than a big glass of red wine is probably a better choice in coping, whether you are pregnant or not.

Gaining Control

It may be that you have not *yet* developed the skill set you need to handle the challenges posed by your pregnancy, but you *can* learn what to do. First, let's take a look at what has worked for you in the past. When things have gotten uncomfortable or out of hand, how have you regained control? Believe it or not, you can adapt this coping mechanism to your pregnancy. Please fill in the chart below to demonstrate your triggers and past effective coping skills.

Situation	How I Gained Control
Parents' divorce	*Talked to friends whose parents were divorced, kept a journal, spoke to the school guidance counselor, started running*

If you are struggling to come up with any ways of gaining control or only have one idea, don't worry. I'll give you the tools you need to face some of the most common challenges of pregnancy and find the best way for you to cope. Experiment with what works for you. You may try one technique at one time and another later in your pregnancy. You may find that you have a favorite technique that consistently works best for you. Whatever works, go for it.

Write It Out

James Pennebaker, a professor of psychology at the University of Texas, has done research into the healing properties of journaling and writing. His work is incredible. He has found that when difficult or traumatic events happen, they tend to stay frozen in time in our minds. Talking about these events only makes us relive them, but his research has shown that writing about these events can have an astonishing healing and cathartic effect on physical and emotional health. Students who wrote about emotionally intense events from their lives for twenty minutes a day for four days became less depressed, were healthier, had better immune functioning, and got better grades. Asthma patients who write about traumas breathe more easily; arthritis patients have better range of motion. There is something incredibly powerful about getting past difficulties down on paper.

I'm not talking here about keeping a sweet baby journal where you note the details of doctors' appointments and the progression of your pregnancy. While that is a wonderful keepsake to have, it is not the same as writing or journaling about your feelings or thoughts as you go through your pregnancy. When you write this kind of journal, it is for venting. It is also for your eyes only, so you can let loose. Something about writing down what you are feeling and thinking definitely provides a release. It's as if those negative thoughts and emotions were rattling around in your brain, gaining momentum, and crowding out your other thoughts, but when you get them down on paper, you have captured them so you can more effectively defuse them or take action as needed. I really don't mean to be disgusting here, but it can be similar to feeling better after throwing up or having awful stomach cramps go away after going to the bathroom. If difficult things have happened to you, getting them down on paper serves as a true catharsis.

Keep in mind that this writing is for no one other than yourself. It's like a letter you would write to someone who has angered you or wronged you but that you would never send. The research shows that the most effective way is to write it by hand, not type. You can keep it or delete it or destroy it. But before you get rid of it, make sure you reread what you wrote, because you can gain considerable insight by reading it all after you have finished. Writing and then destroying the letter can be liberating. But the true benefit lies in writing down and then rereading your thoughts and feelings. Reading and reflecting on what you have written can lead to your putting two and two together and gaining a better understanding of your situation as well as how you are feeling about it and why. It can also diminish some of the power that negative thoughts might have. Seeing it in black and white allows you to examine the truth of the statement in a way that you can't when it is spinning around in your head.

You might also find that you understand another person's actions after writing about them. A family member once said something to me that was incredibly hurtful. I sat down and wrote about my anger and frustration. I included what he had said and how I interpreted it. By the end of twenty minutes, I had figured out why he said it, and although I couldn't forgive him on the spot, understanding why he had said it made it much easier for me to move past it.

Some studies have shown that editing and rewriting your own narrative can have positive results. A study at Duke University showed that when freshmen who were initially struggling with grades and college were given information that what they were experiencing was fairly typical, they were able to rewrite their stories to reflect an adjustment to the rigors of college. Those students went on to improve their grades and had a low dropout rate. The control group who did not receive any information on the typical challenges of college and did not rewrite their stories had a much higher dropout rate.[1]

Writing can help you review, reflect on, and revise your thoughts, feelings, and experiences during your pregnancy.

Mindfulness

Mindfulness is simply being aware, being in the moment. As a long-standing chocoholic, here's how I teach my patients mindfulness. I hand them a Hershey's Kiss and ask them to peel off the wrapper and eat the chocolate mindfully. They will carefully unwrap the foil and either nibble the Kiss or allow it to slowly dissolve in their mouths. Then I ask them, "What does it say on the little paper wrapper?" Most people hadn't noticed. (Do you know what that little piece of paper says?) When you eat a Kiss mindfully, you realize a lot of things you would not have noticed before. How much noise it makes when you peel it, the shape of the aluminum wrapper, how the chocolate really tastes, how it feels melting in your mouth. And yes, what the little piece of paper says, which is "Kisses, Kisses, Kisses."

Sometimes, when your mind is spinning out of control over the what-ifs of pregnancy or you are feeling so down in the dumps that you can't shake the doldrums, it can be healing to immerse yourself in the moment. Now, it may seem that immersing yourself in the what-ifs or the "why mes" will only make things worse, but you will be surprised how the opposite is the case. There are many ways to be mindful. You can take a walk mindfully, cook something mindfully, take a bath, make love, or simply breathe. The key is to focus your mind on what is going on around and within you, rather than on your ever-chattering (and often negative) thoughts.

Walking Mindfully

Here is how to put yourself fully in the moment when you take a mindful walk. Ask yourself the following questions:

- *What do I hear?* Really listen. Birds? Dogs barking? Honking cars?
- *What do I feel?* Be aware of the sensation of the sun on your skin; a breeze in your hair; the crunch of snow beneath your feet.
- *What do I smell?* Are there flowers? Aromas of your neighbor's dinner cooking? Freshly cut grass?
- *What do I see?* Actively see what is around you. How would you describe to someone else, in great detail, what you can see? Try to notice a new detail on something you have passed by before—on the houses, buildings, trees, or cars you walk by.

Eating Mindfully

When you eat mindfully, you can draw on the same questions you used while walking:

- *What do I hear?* The crunch of the apple as I bite into it.
- *What do I feel?* The round shape of the cool fruit in my hand.
- *What do I smell?* The aroma of fresh apple.
- *What do I see?* The pale apple flesh in contrast with the skin.
- *What do I taste?* Sweet, cool, crisp.

Eating mindfully can be wonderfully relaxing under normal circumstances. I can make a good chocolate chip cookie last fifteen minutes. However, I know, particularly in the first trimester, that focusing on taste can have negative consequences, but you can turn that around by imagining a taste that makes you feel good and that isn't a trigger for nausea. So, for example, try eating a bowl of tart lemon sorbet. Or a bowl of salty chips. But take one bite at a time, and focus on the experience of each bite. Pay attention to taste, texture, and temperature.

Here are some additional situations/experiences that my patients have used to increase their mindfulness:

- Sitting in the backyard watching birds at a bird feeder.
- Listening to music, which means listening to every note, not letting your mind wander and the music fade into the background.
- Being outside with the sun on your face (don't forget sunscreen!).
- Making a salad. Focusing on the colors of the vegetables, the sound they make when sliced, the patterns they make in the salad bowl.

Mindfulness is a fabulous skill set. Often women are so focused on the baby or the physical discomfort of pregnancy that they do not experience the here and now of their lives. They become caught up with what will happen to them once the baby is born and miss really experiencing the pregnancy itself. Mindfulness is the perfect counter to this impatience. It is miraculous to have a baby inside you; you can gain access to that miracle by being mindful.

Being with Baby

Just sit and be with your baby—feel it move inside you. It's amazing! People who have never been pregnant can't understand or appreciate what it is like to feel a life inside you. Personally, I thought it was the coolest thing ever! I loved feeling my daughters kick and swim around, even at 2:00

a.m. in what felt like the Olympic trials for baby-bump gymnastics. You may even miss feeling it after the baby is born. Or wish you had paid more attention. I know I did. The only reason I ever considered having a third baby was that I missed the feeling of having a baby inside me.

To be honest, pregnancy is a lot easier (and lasts less time) than taking care of your baby. (Don't worry, taking care of a baby is pretty awesome.) When you focus solely on the results, you miss the process. When you worry about what will come after, and what will be at the end of pregnancy, you miss out on the nine months leading up to the birth. Especially if you focus only on the worries. So be mindful of the special and miraculous aspects of your pregnancy; trust me, the cup really is at least half full.

Self-Nurturance

Most women are typically super conscious of "getting through" the pregnancy, but they need to self-nurture to fully experience their pregnancy. Because self-nurturance doesn't come automatically or easily to most people, you need to determine what will help you in any given situation. I am not talking about being selfish; I am talking self-care. Being selfish means doing for yourself at the expense of others (eating all the chocolate chip cookies), while self-nurturance means doing for yourself in conjunction with the needs of others (buying a box of chocolate chip cookies to satisfy a craving but also sharing them with your family). It can be uncomfortable for most women to meet their own needs, but because it gets much harder once you become a mom, now is actually the best time to learn how to care compassionately for yourself.

When you are faced with fear, sadness, or discomfort, ask yourself, "What will make me feel . . .

. . . Happier?"

. . . Healthier?"

. . . More energetic?"

Then go and do one of those things. Or, make a promise to yourself that you will do it once you get home from work or before the day is done. So, for example, if you are really dragging one day and don't have an opportunity for a nap, take ten minutes for a quick walk around the block or call your funniest friend or indulge in watching your favorite soap or sitcom. You know yourself better than anyone, so begin to think about what works for you to help yourself feel better; even keep a list on your smart phone, your tablet, or a sticky note by your computer, and when you need it, go for it!

During your pregnancy, it is important to take the time to take care of yourself. It's a lesson that you must learn while you are pregnant because if you don't take care of yourself later, you won't be able to care effectively for anyone else. Especially your brand-new baby!

Using Self-Nurturance Throughout Your Pregnancy

Many of my patients have busy lives. They may be juggling work, home, and family obligations and don't always take time for themselves. I think it is important for you to take time every day for your mind to *stop* and just be. Ask yourself every morning, "What do I need?" It won't be the same every day, and the first time you ask yourself this question, it might take you some time to come up with an answer. As time goes on and you get more in tune with your needs, you will come to the answer more quickly.

First trimester: You are likely focused on your body (nausea, fatigue, need to pee). Take time to make yourself more comfortable physically. One way to self-nurture is to figure out how to control your nausea (both the things that make you feel nauseated and those that might help calm nausea). Typical triggers for nausea include coffee, fish, and meat. But be careful in how you go about nurturing yourself. One of my patients could only eat cold sliced turkey during her first trimester. So she decided that she would nurture herself by roasting a turkey. The smell of the roasting turkey filled the house, and that soon became a problem. The smell started to make her feel ill, so when her husband came home that night, she not only was hiding in the attic to escape the smell but refused to come down until he threw out the offending bird!

Good tastes for keeping nausea at bay are typically citrus and salty. That's why so many people recommend saltine crackers during the first months of pregnancy. Crackers usually don't trigger the nausea reflex and can help you avoid having an empty stomach. Some women have found relief by sniffing half of a cut lemon, sucking on a peppermint, or eating ginger.

Second trimester: Although you may not feel like it, exercise (with your OB's permission) is the perfect antidote to the constipation you may experience at this stage in your pregnancy. If you walk with a friend, you get two benefits for the price of one: exercise plus social support.

Try taking time out of your day for some mini relaxation techniques (see below and appendix I). Physically, you may find yourself short of breath as your baby takes up more room in your body, but if you feel comfortable focusing on your breath for short periods of time, "minis" can really help.

A Good Breath of Calming Air: A Mini Relaxation

Close your eyes and take a couple of slow deep breaths (or as deep as you can take with someone camping out just below your lungs). Say the number "ten" to yourself as you inhale, and then slowly exhale. For the next breath, say the number "nine" to yourself, and then slowly exhale. Do this until you get down to "zero." Try opening your eyes. Feel any more relaxed?

Or as you take slow comfortable breaths, count from one to four as you inhale, and then count from four to one as you exhale. Do that five times.

Third trimester: Most women experience more physical symptoms at this point in their pregnancies: heartburn, leg cramps, interrupted sleep. (I'll cover sleep in the next chapter.) Let your OB know about any uncomfortable physical symptoms that are persistent. For heartburn, try to identify what foods trigger it (most commonly, spicy foods, caffeine, and acidic foods like citrus) and avoid eating them, especially in the evening. An antacid, liquid or chewable, can provide relief. Gentle massage can do wonders for leg cramps or an aching back. There is actually some terrific research on the efficacy of partner massage on depressive symptoms. Ask your partner to massage away!

Tools, Approaches

In addition to coping with the physical effects of pregnancy, you will need to develop methods for coping with its mental and emotional aspects. Again, trying different approaches for different issues can work, or find one approach that you love and works best for you in all situations. There are some crossovers here because the physical and the mental can be so closely tied together. Exercise can help body and mind and is a great healer. Studies have shown that exercise can actually reduce stress and depression better than medication or counseling.

Some approaches, like cognitive behavior therapy, may require that you find a therapist to teach you the method. But once you know how to do it, you can use it under any circumstances. CBT is a psychological approach to dealing with emotions and behaviors. It focuses on problem solving and helps to develop skills that can work in any situation. CBT can be effective throughout your pregnancy (and afterward too). Most of what goes through your head at any stage of pregnancy is cognitive distortion—meaning inaccurate negative thoughts and emotions. CBT will help you to work with what you are thinking and feeling and help you to gain a different perspective. There is a large amount of evidence that CBT is equal to or better than antidepressant medication in treating mild to moderate symptoms. Recent psychiatric research concludes that CBT is the optimal first-line treatment for depression. Relapse rates are lower for CBT than for medication, and CBT is more cost-effective than medication. Also, there are no negative side effects from CBT and thus no risk to your baby.[2] We all have automatic thoughts that play over and over in our heads, and because negative emotions seem to be common during pregnancy, it's not surprising that CBT can be so helpful.

Other approaches that you can turn to when you are feeling sad, anxious, or depressed include the following:

Acupuncture—If you choose acupuncture, be sure the practitioner is knowledgeable about treating a pregnant woman. Acupuncture is safe to use during pregnancy and is an effective treatment for nausea and vomiting, as well as depression and anxiety.

Exercise—As I have said before, exercise will do more for you than anything else. It is a happy pill that's free and has no side effects. If you stay fit, or work to become fit, you can decrease anxiety and depression and feel more in control. But make sure you have your OB's okay before starting.

Taking a walk in nature with friends can boost your mood. "Group nature walks are linked with significantly lower depression, less perceived stress, and enhanced mental health and well-being, according to the study conducted by the University of Michigan, with partners from De Montfort University, James Hutton Institute, and Edge Hill University in the United Kingdom."[3]

You can be fit and pregnant at the same time. Labor will be faster, and you will get your body back more quickly after the baby is born.

Light Therapy—Exposure to particular light waves can serve to elevate mood. This therapy is often used for people who have seasonal affective disorder (SAD). A light box emits light that is similar to outdoor light, countering the lack of sunlight experienced in fall and winter when SAD is most likely to occur. Speak to your doctor or therapist to see if this might be a recommended approach. There is a potential for light therapy to trigger mania in those with bipolar disorder, so please check with your doctor first.

Massage—Massage is wonderful for relieving aches and pains, but when you are pregnant, be sure to get a massage from someone who is familiar with working with pregnant women and is skilled in prenatal massage.

Meditation—You may be familiar with meditation, which is a technique that allows you to focus your thoughts to achieve peace and perspective. The basic idea of meditation is to focus on a word or phrase and repeat it silently to yourself in rhythm with your breath. So, for example, many of my patients choose to use "peace and calm" or "the Lord is my shepherd" or "breathing in peace and calm, breathing out tension and anxiety." Try it for ten to twenty minutes on a daily basis. The more you do it, the less your mind will wander.

Fran, who now has fraternal twins, faced some challenges in her pregnancy. After seven cycles of IVF and three miscarriages, she became pregnant with her boys. As the pregnancy progressed and the boys grew, she had trouble breathing and experienced swelling, along with rapid weight gain. Sleep was elusive because she would wake up in the night, not only to pee, but because her "mind was racing" with concerns for her health and the babies' health. For three weeks prior to delivery, she was hospitalized with pre-eclampsia. In all that she went through, she found value in meditation and used it throughout her pregnancy. "I did it every day. I had a podcast that I listened to for my whole pregnancy. I don't do it now, but wish I could get back to it."

Supplements—Women are advised to take a prenatal vitamin prior to getting pregnant (if possible) and then throughout the pregnancy. There are hundreds of other supplements available in your grocery store, health food store, local pharmacy, and online. Please be careful about what you take. There are thousands of claims made about supplements, and because they aren't regulated by the Food and Drug Administration (FDA), almost none of those claims are true. You may see something promoted on the Web or on the news, but I'd exercise caution here. Ask your OB or nurse-midwife before taking any supplement other than a prenatal vitamin.

There are some preliminary data on the use of omega-3s for the treatment of depression during pregnancy, but the results are not definitive. When it comes to anything that you take during pregnancy, I would recommend you follow the advice of your obstetrician.

Yoga—There are many forms of yoga, and prenatal yoga classes (taught by an experienced instructor) can give you a gentle workout and allow you to turn off your mind for a little while. Many of my patients love going to a prenatal yoga class because it gives them a chance to partake in an effective relaxation technique, keeps them fit and toned, and provides social support by enabling them to hang out with other pregnant women.

Yoga and a swim class were excellent ways for Carrie to stay active and find community. "My yoga instructor was really incredible. I told her I was pregnant (eight weeks), and she gave me protective positions to do that were easy for me and safe for the baby. I also joined a prenatal swim class and met a woman who was six weeks ahead of me, and we became close. She was a lifeline in a big way. We jokingly called the class 'The Whale Class'; we laughed together, and it was a bonding time and was really nice. A number of us had infertility stories, and it felt like a safe space to share my own story."

All of these approaches can help you to self-nurture, relax, safely express your emotions, let go of perfectionism. If you take a group class, you can either gain some social support from an instructor who understands what you are going through or connect with other pregnant women who may be experiencing similar physical and emotional symptoms to yours.

Coping with Change

One of the first mind shifts I encourage my patients to take is to acknowledge that their lives will change and that for the most part it will be for the better. The other side of that coin is that it is *normal* to feel some regret about your perceived losses and feel ambivalent about being pregnant. Any time you make a major decision or make a change in your life, you will likely have second thoughts. Ambivalence is normal and healthy. You will always wonder, what if . . . It's human nature. I wanted to be pregnant with both of my children and had wanted to be a mom my whole life. But I remember about ten weeks into my first pregnancy feeling so sick and tired of being sick and tired that I told my mother I thought I had made the wrong decision. She basically told me to suck it up, that the suffering would be worth it, and you know what? She was right. But please don't feel guilty if you find yourself occasionally resenting being pregnant.

I also encourage you to keep in mind that pregnancy itself is time limited and you won't feel like this forever. It can *feel* as if you will be throwing up forever, but it will come to an end. It can *feel* as if you will always be bigger than your pre-pregnancy self, but you will lose weight. Ambivalence, guilt, and fear are so very common during pregnancy, and they don't mean that you will be a bad mom or that you are causing some harm to your baby by questioning your condition. What they really mean is that your hormones are higher than you have ever experienced before in your life. They mean that you are distracted, anxious, and tired and it's hard to think clearly. Feeling ambivalent does not indicate some flaw in you; it's normal and largely due to your raging hormones and your tired brain running amok.

Medication During Pregnancy

You should know that I have, on many occasions, recommended that a pregnant patient see a psychiatrist in order to get medication to treat her symptoms of depression and/or anxiety. I don't make this recommendation lightly but only when it will be safer for everyone, including the pregnant woman, to do so. A number of psychiatrists specialize in treating women while they are trying to conceive, during pregnancy, and after delivery.

⊰⊱

Making a Decision to Medicate

Eliza is a mother of two who has a personal and family history of depression; both she and her father experienced bouts of depressive symptoms. With her first, she says she had expected pregnancy to be "everything sweet, lovey-dovey, and romantic." Instead, she says it was "so anxiety producing! When I found out I was pregnant, even after years of trying, I totally freaked out. I was *so* anxious for the first three months, and there was a lack of control when this happens. I had fears about what to do, how I would cope with having a baby."

For her second pregnancy, she went on Prozac to ward off anxiety. "I felt that because the anxiety was so bad with the first pregnancy, I had to do something proactive with the second. I felt I couldn't be in the same situation I was with the first pregnancy. I also felt I couldn't let my first child down. We talked about our risk, and it felt like an okay decision to go on the medication. I don't regret it at all and wish I'd been on medication for the first pregnancy as well."

Now, she says, "exercise, meditation, and medication work for me."

Because I don't know you, and can't treat you in person, I can't make any blanket recommendations about medication in this book. If you are experiencing symptoms of depression or anxiety, it is important that you consult with your OB or a mental health professional about taking any medications whether by prescription or over the counter. That being said, the information below should help you when you have these conversations and aid you in coming to a more informed decision regarding medication during *your* pregnancy.

The most commonly prescribed class of antidepressants is an SSRI. SSRI stands for "selective serotonin reuptake inhibitor." SSRIs block cells in your brain from admitting serotonin—a chemical that affects mood. Common SSRIs include Prozac, Zoloft, Paxil, and Lexapro. If you experienced depression or mood issues prior to your pregnancy, you might have been prescribed an SSRI. You may want to resume taking an SSRI for depression or a mood issue now that you are pregnant, but you should do so only if you consult with your OB and prescribing physician.

Until recently, most health-care professionals believed that it was far safer for a depressed pregnant woman to take an SSRI during pregnancy than to experience depressive symptoms. However, recent research has affected the opinions and prescribing recommendations of many. Most pregnant women who take an SSRI during pregnancy will in fact deliver a healthy baby. Up to 13 percent of pregnant women take an antidepressant for all or part of their pregnancy.[4] However, taking an SSRI during pregnancy appears to increase the risk of miscarriage, preterm birth, low birth weight, and health issues with the newborn and is associated with an increased risk of ADD/ADHD and autism.

Medication might be the right approach for your individual circumstances, particularly *if* you have had depression in the past and are at risk for harming yourself in any way (contemplating suicide, not eating, taking drugs). In that case, under a psychiatrist's supervision, taking an SSRI is the safest option for you. *However*, most women don't fall under that category. What I have found about most women who are prescribed medications is the following:

- They have not been evaluated by a mental health professional.
- They do not have *severe* symptoms of depression.

Of the 13 percent of pregnant women taking an SSRI, it is likely that only a small percentage need to continue taking it to keep safe. If a woman is not experiencing an ideal quality of life but is not a danger to herself or the baby, then she should consider pursuing other approaches to treating her depressive symptoms. Unless someone is really at risk, it seems to make sense to try other approaches first. If none of them work, then SSRIs can be prescribed.

Talk to Your Doctor

Before taking any medication, you need to understand the risks and benefits. The best way to do this is to have a conversation with a health professional in order to weigh the pros and cons of different treatments. The first conversation you should have is with your OB, nurse, or midwife. Be honest. If you are holding in negative emotions or thoughts, don't.

Many women feel embarrassed about feeling conflicted or sad when they are pregnant, but it is *so* common. Unload on your OB (your doctor has probably heard it all before, and you won't surprise her); if you don't let her know the truth of what you are thinking and feeling, she won't be able to help you. During your visit, she will be mindful of getting a read on your mood, but she has only so much time in the appointment, so it's up to you to raise the issue with her. She should be able to refer you to an appropriate mental health professional.

✤

Medication May Be Right for You If . . .

- you are miserable with no quality of life and can't imagine getting through the next day
- you have thoughts of harming yourself
- you hate yourself
- your outlook is dark all the time and you can't imagine that ever changing

If you are feeling this way, you may benefit from medication. If you want to hurt yourself or are taking drugs or consuming alcohol, it is urgent that you seek the guidance of a mental health professional or your doctor.

Unless you are severely depressed and can't function, it is worth trying something else for a couple of weeks. If the alternative doesn't work, then you can try medication. You can always revisit the issue, but it is better to start with the least invasive/risky approach.

The research on the non-medication treatment of depressive symptoms in pregnant women indicates that a number of other treatments may well be just as effective. These treatments include CBT and other forms of counseling, exercise, acupuncture, massage, and some forms of light treatment.

A Word on Over-the-Counter Medications

While we all reach for over-the-counter products to help with sleep, discomfort, and other ailments, this should not be so automatic when you are pregnant. There is no compelling information that anything sold over the counter will help you feel less anxious or depressed. In fact, it is best to avoid over-the-counter medications altogether unless your OB says it is okay to take them. Also, please stay away from herbs and supplements other than prenatal vitamins or ones your health-care team specifically recommends. Common herbs that are recommended to decrease anxiety are chamomile, Saint-John's-wort, and lemon balm, but these have not been adequately tested on pregnant women.

You should know that herbs and dietary supplements are not regulated by the FDA. There have been instances of herbs from China that were contaminated with lead and mercury that could have a detrimental effect on your baby. A recent report in *The New York Times* states, "The New York State attorney general's office accused four major retailers of selling fraudulent and potentially dangerous herbal supplements and demanded that they remove the products from their shelves."[5]

Therapy

How do you know if you need a therapist? This may be one of those times when, if you think you'd like to talk to a therapist, you should probably investigate further. If you are depressed or anxious and have decided against taking medication, then you will need someone to talk to who can help you navigate your way through your pregnancy and teach you how to effectively cope with your feelings and emotions. If you don't have someone you can speak with easily, if you don't feel as if you have the support of your family or friends, you will find that having someone to talk to (who isn't judging you) can be wonderful. Even if you could simply use a boost or a fine-tuning of your coping skills or need a sounding board for what you are thinking and experiencing during your pregnancy, a therapist can fit the bill.

Choosing a Therapist

To find a therapist, ask your OB, nurse, or midwife if he or she has any referrals. Many psychiatrists do not practice as therapists anymore, so ask about psychologists, social workers, and licensed mental health counselors. It is important that you find someone who is familiar and comfortable working with pregnant women (remember, the signs of depression are the same as the symptoms of early pregnancy and you want to work with someone who knows this). Ask. Ask about his or her experience or comfort level if there are particular circumstances of your pregnancy that you would like the therapist to be familiar with—pregnancy as a result of fertility treatments, high-risk pregnancy, and so on. You want to be sure that the therapist has experience that will be relevant to your situation. And remember, you want to have a good fit so you will feel comfortable unburdening yourself. A therapist who is great for one person might not be ideal for another, so spend some time evaluating the therapist. I am a huge believer in chemistry between you and your therapist. Talk to him or her over the phone for a few minutes before making an appointment. You can tell a lot about someone via a brief chat. And if you don't feel comfortable after a session or two, find someone else. I like to believe that I am a good therapist, but I have to say there are times when a perfectly lovely patient comes to see me and we just don't click. It is far better for her to find someone else than to continue to see me.

Red Flags

Working with a therapist can be incredibly rewarding, but keep alert for potential red flags that may indicate that the therapist is not for you. If a therapist shares too much personal information (an anecdote or two is okay; intimate details of her life are not), or if he is an alarmist and talking to him feels more like adding gasoline to the fire, rather than turning down the flame, you are not being helped in the way you need. If you feel a lot worse after therapy, and those bad feelings continue, it's not a good fit. Keep in mind that sometimes therapy can stir up some negative emotions, but in general you want to feel good about going to therapy and feel as if you have been making progress when you leave.

The therapist should be empathetic and supportive and give you ideas or strategies on how to cope. You should leave your visit feeling empowered and that the person knows what he or she is talking about. You should want to go back. You should be helped to tap into or develop the skills that will enable you to feel better. The therapist should be an active, not passive, listener. She should be a warm, sympathetic sounding board. She should be reassuring but savvy. A therapist should also be open to the idea of talking with your family. A therapist can serve as a third party to help your partner better understand your situation or mediate if there is an issue between you and your partner. I have sat down with partners, parents, in-laws, and so on, and sometimes feel more like a mediator than a psychologist. I actually said to the husband of one of my patients last week that the only two words he was allowed to utter in the delivery room were "Yes, dear." Drastic, I know, but he needed to hear it.

$\propto$

A Note to Partners of Pregnant Women

It is important for you to understand that your partner's complaints are legit. Pregnancy can be exhausting, and she needs your support when she feels nauseated, tired, or upset. Your little baby has taken over her body. She may already be well into the baby more than you are, she may be too tired or too nauseated for sex (or anything), she may pass out on the couch during the six o'clock news, and she may be jealous of the attention the baby is getting; heck, *you* may be jealous of the attention the baby is getting. There is a lot going on in her body and her mind, and one of your jobs is to support her to feel better. Trust me, doubting her is not an option. If she says she feels bad, take her at her word.

Pregnancy can be stressful and bring on a host of physical and emotional discomforts. However, there are plenty of things you can do on your own or with the help of a professional to combat your negative thoughts and feelings and deal with them effectively. The more you can reduce your stress and anxiety, the better you will feel and the better it will be for your baby.

Chapter 4

The Pregnant Brain

Most of my patients ask me about "pregnancy brain" or, as it is sometimes called, "momnesia." In the U.K., it is called porridge brain! It is the phenomenon that seems to make pregnant women more forgetful than usual. In fact, I was once asked to look into the available studies and write an article about "pregnant brain," so I am in effect a published author on the topic. Research shows that in the first and second trimesters pregnant women are actually not any spacier than they were before they conceived; they tend not to think any differently than they did prior to their pregnancy. However, in the third trimester, some studies did find a cognitive shift where women might think more slowly and make more mistakes. Many of my patients report feeling distracted and forgetful. It's understandable; every cell in a woman's body is affected by pregnancy; it's no wonder the mind is too. There is no way you *can't* think differently. But beyond forgetfulness and difficulty with concentration, the biggest shift in thinking I see is women engaging in distorted thinking—essentially negative thoughts that don't reflect reality. Although largely untrue, distorted thinking can add stress, which in turn can raise your anxiety. Anxiety is extremely common during pregnancy. Recent studies suggest that up to 20 percent of women suffer from mood or anxiety disorders during pregnancy.[1]

This is not to say that one should never worry during pregnancy. Apart from the normal "midnight imp" favorites, many pregnant women have real reasons for concern. Most of the pregnant patients I see are not in fact having easy, effortless, happy-go-lucky pregnancies. They have true cause for concern; they might have had a miscarriage or a stillbirth, or there might be a family history of birth defects, among other issues. But even in these situations, in almost every case, their odds for having a healthy baby are huge. It's my job to help these women acknowledge that their worry is to be expected, but to put their concerns into perspective and to enjoy their pregnancy as much as possible.

When You Worry

Jenny, now the mother of a toddler, had a stillbirth with her first pregnancy. Her first pregnancy had been uneventful, which caused her much concern with her second. She was worried throughout her second pregnancy and felt *very* stressed. "I knew I wanted to have children," she said, "but being pregnant was frightening because of the chance of stillbirth. I was scared all the time; I felt like I was holding my breath. It was so *very* stressful!" A single mom, Jenny had lots of emotional support from her own mother, and that helped to ease her anxiety. In addition, she says, "I didn't want to burden anyone, so I went to a therapist—a professional. I thought it would be better to talk to someone who had insight and understood my situation."

Margo, mother of a six-month-old, had a miscarriage in her first pregnancy. She says, "I worried about having that happen again. Every week I felt I was getting closer to safety. I was scared to take any risks (not even a sip of wine). I felt very guarded until fifteen weeks went by. Pregnancy was an emotional roller coaster. I was mostly joyful, but there were tears (and I was that way postpartum too). Now if I cry, my husband asks me if I'm pregnant."

Worry isn't necessarily surprising if you have a history of miscarriage or if you are concerned about a family medical history of a genetic condition. Don't worry about worrying! The important thing is not to let worry consume you. Talk to your OB or nurse-midwife, seek information about your concerns from a reliable resource. Find ways to take a break from worry and engage with your partner, your friends, and your family.

Coping with Change

People, in general, are resistant to change. Change, even brought about by positive events, can bring anxious thoughts. One of the best-known scales to measure stress is called the Holmes and Rahe Stress Scale. It assigns a numerical ranking to a range of stressful events. Most of the top ten are negative, such as the death of a spouse, divorce, or a jail term, but many of the events are positive. Marriage is number 7, and marital reconciliation is number 9. Pregnancy is number 12, well ahead of financial challenges and the death of a close friend.

In pregnancy, everything is changing. You may be happy about being pregnant, but adapting to pregnancy and impending motherhood can lead to a lot of stressful thoughts. Being anxious pulls your attention in multiple directions or can distract you from the task at hand, so it's easy to feel fuzzy and slow-witted. Additionally, when they are pregnant, women's anxious thoughts tend toward catastrophizing, and this can be especially troubling in the middle of the night. The worry feels so real, so scary, and so awful. The same thought in the middle of the day may not seem as dire, but that midnight imp will come to plague you and push your thoughts into negative territory:

I'm not going to be able to handle work if I have a baby.
I'll never get my body back.

I'm going to be a terrible mom.
My partner/spouse doesn't find me attractive.
We'll never be financially secure again.
Something is wrong with the baby.
If something is wrong, I won't be able to handle it.
The baby will permanently (negatively) affect my
  relationship with my partner/spouse.
What if the baby has a birth defect and it's my fault?
I don't know if I will love the baby.
My partner and I will never have fun again as a couple.
What if I hate being a mother?
What if the baby is colicky?
What if I pass on some family disease or disorder to
  my baby?
I'll never lose the baby weight.
My partner/spouse will never be attracted to me again.
I'll never look good again.
What if the baby cries all the time?
My partner will be repulsed by my pregnant body and how
  I look afterward.
We can't afford a baby.

Do any of these sound familiar? These are some of the concerns that have worried my patients (and me! The midnight imp visited me a lot when I was pregnant). Everyone worries about her baby, her partner, and her future. And, within reason, worry can help you to troubleshoot for potential issues and prepare you to face them. However, the kind of distorted thinking that keeps you up at night is often driven by anxiety and fear and not based in reality.

During pregnancy, it can feel as if your body is out of control, your mind is racing, you are faced with great unknowns, and people treat you differently. The information you receive from friends, family, or the Internet can be out of balance and contradictory. You might feel as if you live in two extremes of either perfect or awful. As you internalize what you see, hear, and read about pregnancy, your brain becomes like a tape recorder that is set to filter out the positive. Consequently, anything positive you hear can be misinterpreted or twisted to be put in a more negative light. If someone says that you are carrying well, you may think to yourself that he or she is just being kind and can't say out loud that you look like a whale.

In fact, the thoughts running around in your brain are roughly 90 percent negative and largely untrue. Nobody is as nasty to you as your own mind. Your mind can be your own worst enemy—sending you spinning into catastrophic thoughts, berating yourself for minor (or imagined) transgressions, and creating scenarios where you always come out on the losing side.

⨯

Cognitive Distortions

David Burns, an adjunct clinical professor emeritus in the Department of Psychiatry and Behavioral Sciences at the Stanford University School of Medicine and the author of *Feeling Good: The New Mood Therapy*, identified the various forms cognitive distortions can take, including all-or-nothing thinking (everything is either all good or all bad) and personalization (everything is all your fault).

Essentially, cognitive distortion colors your thought process so that you see only the negative in most situations, take blame for all things, or take no responsibility for your role in any given situation. If this sounds like you, his workbook, *The Feeling Good Handbook*, is a must-read.

David Burns's research showed that your mind can skew your perception of reality, and it does it all the time. It's a good thing that the power of your mind is such that it can be turned around to be your best ally. The way you tap into that positive power is to challenge the negative thoughts by asking, is what I am saying to myself *logical* and *true*? As you will see from the following exercise, it's not. Our tape-recorder brain plays the same negative untrue thoughts over and over. If you hear it often enough, you begin to believe that it must be true, even if the thoughts and perceptions are solely created in your own mind. We become so used to these thoughts that we never stop and actually confront or challenge them. But from now on, by using something called cognitive restructuring, you will be equipped to take on those thoughts and turn them around.

Cognitive Restructuring

It is very common to engage in negative, catastrophic thinking—especially at night. When you are busy throughout the day, these kinds of thoughts don't have an opportunity to break in and take hold. But when you get up to go to the bathroom in the middle of the night (again), suddenly your rational brain is taken over and that little devil causes havoc with your thoughts. It's okay to think things that are not true or logical (playing at being an astronaut when you were a little girl, imagining winning the lottery now), but you have to challenge them when they are contributing to your stress, anxiety, or depression. In most cases, it's your emotions that are altering the truth of the statements. What you need to do is to reframe these thoughts to make them factual.

Recognizing Distorted Thinking by Using Cognitive Restructuring

There is a very helpful technique that can help you to rein in those runaway thoughts and cut your catastrophic thinking down to size. It requires writing and reflecting on those negative, distorted thoughts, so you might want to keep a small pen and notebook by the side of your bed so you can write down the intrusive thought, promise yourself that you will tackle it in the morning, and get back to your much-needed sleep. You can do the same thing in the light of day. Monitor your repetitive thoughts, jot them down, and tackle them when you have a few minutes for reflection.

The Four Questions

First, write down the thought. Then ask yourself the following questions:

1. Does this thought contribute to my stress?
2. Where did I learn this thought? These thoughts usually come from something someone said to you in the past (Mom, is that you?)—or is it your fear speaking?
3. Is this a logical thought?
4. Is this thought true?

Once you have evaluated your thought for truth and logic, you can restructure the thought so that the emotional aspect has been removed and it has become a true and logical statement.

EXAMPLE:

I will never get my body back!

1. Does this thought contribute to my stress?

Yes, you can see yourself getting larger and can't see how that big belly and hips will all go away after the baby is born.

2. Where did I learn this thought?

This is most likely FEAR talking. (Has your OB, or anyone else, said to you that you will never get your body back?)

3. Is this a logical thought?

No, it's not. Lots of people lose the pregnancy weight and get back into their skinny jeans. Besides, it's not logical to say "never." Yes, some part of you may not be the same (your breasts may be bigger or smaller, and there may be subtle shifts in your body), but it will still be your body, and there are many things you can do to keep it healthy.

4. Is this thought true?

No. It's not true, because you don't know what will happen. If you are eating relatively responsibly (not mashed potatoes and ice cream every day), your pregnancy will not permanently affect your ability to be at a healthy weight and look terrific.

It is challenging to gain weight and see your body changing. And the way a woman's body reacts in pregnancy unfolds differently for everyone. When confronting change now, or anticipating change in the future, one must embrace realistic expectations.

You can restructure the original thought to one that *is* true and logical, such as:

I don't know what will happen. If I eat as well as possible and exercise, I will get my body back sooner rather than later.

This statement is not only true, it is not emotionally loaded. It doesn't have the telltale word "never" and puts you more in control of what will come next.

$\div$

I'm going to hate being a mother!

1. Does this thought contribute to my stress?

Yes.

2. Where did I learn this thought?

Perhaps you hated looking after your siblings; perhaps you hated babysitting.

3. Is this a logical thought?

No; you are pregnant, so there must be a piece of you that wants to become a mother. (Worrying about your abilities is actually the first sign that you care and will do your best as a mother.)

4. Is this thought true?

Don't know. If you have never parented before, there is no evidence to say one way or the other.

Keep in mind that parenting your own child is very different from taking care of siblings (it's a different relationship) or babysitting (it's a job). Lots of people don't like babysitting, but they did it to earn money. You cannot determine if you are fit to be a parent based on your babysitting experience. A childhood friend hated babysitting but absolutely loves being a mom. But this fear haunted her during her pregnancy. Being a parent is truly unlike anything you have ever done before. It is one of those rare life events where you can't rely on past experience to guide you.

You can restructure the original thought to one that *is* true and logical, such as:

I'm afraid it is going to be hard to be a mom. I don't know how good a mother I will be. But I look forward to experiencing both the challenges and the joys.

⚭

My partner and I will never have fun together again!

1. Does this thought contribute to my stress?

Yes.

2. Where did I learn this thought?

Other people have said it, and it is your FEAR speaking. (Honestly, people wouldn't have kids if it sucked the fun out of life.)

3. Is this a logical thought?

No, people wouldn't have kids if this were true. Or second kids, for that matter.

4. Is this thought true?

There is no way of knowing if this is true or not. However, parenting a child with your partner has the potential of being lots of fun. It is fun to have kids. Kids make you laugh. There is no one other than your partner who thinks your kids are so amazing. It's great to see all of your kids' firsts. Many people think that having a child brings more joy into life. Yes, it's a different kind of fun, but it's not worse; it's equally as joyful. You will be creating a family history together, as parents and children.

You can restructure the original thought to one that *is* true and logical, such as:

We may not have the kind of couple fun we had before (hot, naked sex), but we'll have family fun. We will have LAUGHTER!

❧

We can't afford a baby!

1. Does this thought contribute to my stress?

Yes.

2. Where did I learn this thought?

This is really just more fear talking. You know that having a baby is expensive.

3. Is this a logical thought?

Hopefully not.

4. Is this thought true?

Hopefully, it's not true.

Kids do cost money, but there are ways to make costs more manageable. You might have to make some sacrifices, but you can be creative. Use hand-me-downs, go out less, or take advantage of activities your city or town or local attractions have to offer free to residents.

You can restructure the original thought to one that *is* true and logical, such as:

We're going to have to live a bit differently to save money so we can support our child. But that is going to be okay.

❧

Cognitive restructuring allows you to take the time to evaluate the thoughts that are contributing to your stress, hold them up to a standard of truth and/or logic, and see where they might be leading you astray.

If you go through this process with any of your concerns, and you answer yes to a "Is it logical or true?" question, then you need to act on it. If one of your negative thoughts has truth in it and that truth can lead to a negative outcome for you or your baby, you need to investigate further and seek help to resolve the situation. Thus, for example, if your negative thought is "I am not bringing my baby into a safe home" and that is a logical and/or true statement, you need to move to a safe place, for both of you.

Self-Talk and Intuition

Another form of self-talk is intuition. It's that small voice inside you or that gut feeling that you can have about a situation or when you are faced with making a decision. On paper, something may look great, but if there is an aspect to it that tells you to be cautious, that's your intuition at work. I'm a scientist, but I am also a big believer in trusting your gut. I think it is important to take your instincts and feelings seriously. If you have a concern, it is better to call your doctor than to kick yourself later. That is what your medical team is there for, and they have probably already heard this, or a similar concern from other patients. If you can't shake a thought that is keeping you up at night, perspective from someone else (and not the Internet) may be in order. Talk it over with your spouse or a friend. Write it down, and bring the question with you to your next doctor's appointment. Use the trustworthy resources that are available to you.

Positive self-talk is another technique that I teach my patients and that you can use to silence that inner critic or the voice that keeps you up at night questioning your abilities to do anything right—including having a healthy pregnancy and being a mom.

Stop, Breathe, Reflect, and Choose

When an intrusive or negative thought pops up:

Stop—Visualize a stop sign

Breathe—Slow down, take a few slow breaths

Reflect—Ask, "What is really going on here?"

Choose—Make the choice to do something that you know will make you feel better. Try to restructure the thought, reframe the idea, take a walk, talk to your partner, have a cup of tea, or call the doctor. Knowing you have a choice increases your sense of control and will make you feel less anxious.

For example, let's say you wake up in the middle of the night to go to the bathroom and when you get back to bed you can't fall asleep because you have a little bit of heartburn. Then you start thinking about it. You've read that everyone gets heartburn, but you've never had it before so you *think* it might be heartburn, but what if it is something else? What if there is something terribly wrong with you?

What if there is something terribly wrong with the baby? First, it is always a good idea to mention any symptoms to your doctor because even if you've heard that it's common in pregnancy, your doctor should be kept apprised of what is going on in your particular pregnancy. Second, it's probably just run-of-the-mill heartburn, but you need to get some sleep, so here are some things you can do to get your rest and put a plan in place to investigate the symptom and resolve your worry.

[Stop] Picture that stop sign. Sit quietly.

[Breathe] Do some mini relaxation techniques. Some simple deep belly breathing that really fills your lungs and then exhaling completely, done slowly, can bring some calm. You can count slowly, backward from a hundred. If you know some meditation techniques, you can do them. (See appendix I for some exercises.)

[Reflect] You can journal about your fear. Writing your thoughts down can capture them for you in a way that will allow you to address them directly, rather than leaving them as an amorphous fear.

[Choose] You can write down your worry and call the doctor in the morning. Look up your doctor's approved list of over-the-counter products. If antacids are on the list, take one and see how you feel.

[Choose] You can wake up your partner and talk it out. It will be helpful for your partner if you are clear about what you need: "I am going to tell you something, and you are not going to solve it or offer solutions; you are going to give me a hug."

❧

Partner Assistance

Write down ten to twelve things that can make you feel better when you are stressed or down. The list is up to your personal taste: a hug, a bouquet of flowers, a funny movie, a foot rub, or whatever works for you. Give the list to your partner so he knows what to do to help you the next time you are feeling anxious or upset. Having the list in hand will make your partner feel better because he will know exactly what to do to help you.

Trust me, he worries that he won't know how to help you or that he will do something that makes you feel worse. Men tend to be problem solvers. They often offer solutions rather than listening to your concerns. They are simply wired differently. Some men live in fear of making you more upset by whatever they suggest. So the list will help you both. And if you want to be a terrific partner, ask your partner for his own list so you can reciprocate. After all, I can guarantee that you aren't the only one who will get stressed or sad during the forty weeks of your pregnancy.

You can only control what you can control. One of the best approaches to dealing with unknowns is to find the resources for what you need to know. Your OB or nurse-midwife knows a lot about pregnancy and childbirth. Trust that he or she knows more than you (despite your intensive Google searches) and is a valuable resource for you. OBs are always monitoring you when they see you; they look and listen beyond what you say to them, but you can help them by being completely honest and up-front about any symptoms or concerns. This is not the time to hold back out of embarrassment. Help them to help you by making them aware of your personal medical history as well as that of your family. Write down your questions, or make a note of them in your smart phone so you are prepared for your next appointment. When you write things down, you will feel better because you have taken the first step toward making a plan. You are letting go of the problem in order to solve it.

Resources at Your Disposal

- Take advantage of the information available at your doctor's office. If the people in the office can't help you with your particular question or situation, they can refer you to someone who can.
- Talk to your therapist. He or she can help you manage your worry, sadness, or depression.

- Get educated:
  - Take a childbirth class; your OB may recommend one, or check the hospital where you plan to deliver.
  - Take an infant CPR class.
  - Take a breast-feeding class (ask your OB or nurse-midwife for a referral).
  - Take a tour of the maternity ward at your hospital.
- Read books such as *What to Expect When You're Expecting*. But trust books written by credentialed professionals rather than an individual's misery memoir. (See appendix II for other recommendations.)

If you go online, try sites like the American Academy of Pediatrics or others that are not commercially based. (See appendix II.) Be very careful about blogs and chat rooms. As I've mentioned, people who have average or normal experiences tend not to post. Some people will exaggerate or downright lie. Some of what is posted is often retrospective, so it's not accurate. Besides, one person's experience will not be identical to yours.

Benefits of Pregnancy Brain

Your mind can lead you astray during pregnancy and fill your brain with negative thoughts. Thankfully, those thoughts can be turned around with a little attention and refocusing. I do think there are some benefits to the changes in your thought processes that occur during pregnancy. They help you to be more vigilant. Worry can sidetrack you, but it can also keep you aware of what you are eating, doing, and feeling. You have a near-constant reminder that you are responsible for someone else. During pregnancy, the brain gets prepared. Worry and anxiety during pregnancy are like a dress rehearsal for when you have a baby and need to be cautious and watchful for someone who is depending on you for care.

Chapter 5

High-Octane Prenatal Self-Care

WHILE MUCH OF the focus during your pregnancy will be on the baby, it is also important to care for yourself in different ways from before you got pregnant. Self-care will lead to a healthier pregnancy and baby. While it may seem as if it's all about the bump, it is really all about you and how you care for yourself and, in turn, how that benefits your baby. You may already eat well, exercise, and generally care for yourself, but the way you engage in self-care shifts when you are expecting.

On the other hand, some women are great at taking care of the other people in their lives—family, friends, neighbors, and co-workers—but struggle to take care of themselves or to put themselves first. Are you the one who says yes to any volunteer opportunity that comes along? Either out of guilt or out of true enthusiasm? Do you do all the cooking at home? Are you the vacation planner, social secretary, and overall go-to person in your relationships? Many of us enjoy doing all that we do. It is a wonderful quality to want to do the things you love for the people you love and the causes you support. But when you are pregnant, you may need to take off one or two of the many hats you wear and embrace the job of being pregnant. Self-care is good for you and good for your baby.

Self-care is particularly important if you have ever had any struggles with anxiety, depression, or mood disorders. You want to be sure that you have the support you need to keep you healthy in mind and body throughout your pregnancy. It's important to work closely with your health-care professionals to be sure you get the care and attention you need. This also goes for when you have never had any problems with your mood prior to your pregnancy but begin to experience anxiety or depression while pregnant. As I've said previously, it's relatively common to have some anxiety or worry during pregnancy, but if it is getting in the way of your caring for yourself, it's important to ask for help for your sake as well as your baby's. It's like what they tell you on an airplane: If you need to use oxygen, take care of yourself before assisting others.

Quiz
Are You Taking Care of Yourself?

❧

1. **How are you sleeping?**

a. *I sleep like a baby.*

b. *I fall asleep easily, often wake up to pee and am up for a bit, but can fall back to sleep.*

c. *Some nights are okay; some are bad. The lack of sleep is getting to me.*

d. *Not at all. I wake up on and off either to pee or because I am anxious and then can't fall back asleep.*

2. **How is your energy level?**

a. *I've been told that pregnant women get tired, but so far I feel like the Energizer Bunny.*

b. *The afternoons are tough, but after I power through that, I'm okay.*

c. *I'm really tired, but I can still accomplish what I have to get done.*

d. *I'm exhausted all of the time.*

3. Are you eating well?

a. *I know what I shouldn't eat and do eat fruits, vegetables, and whole grains.*

b. *I've memorized the nutrition chapter from* What to Expect When You're Expecting; *I weigh all of my food and have every meal and snack that is recommended.*

c. *I'm pretty much eating what I ate before, but I take a prenatal vitamin.*

d. *I'm eating exactly the way I ate before—chips, soda, sweets. I'm okay, and the baby will be too.*

4. How regularly do you exercise?

a. *I exercise seven days a week without fail.*

b. *I exercise most days as long as I have the energy.*

c. *I take a prenatal yoga class once a week and occasionally take a walk.*

d. *I refer to this as a couch pregnancy.*

Scoring: Give yourself the following points for each answer you circled, then use the chart that follows to determine how stressed you are about being pregnant:

- Score 0 for each A answer.
- Score 1 for each B answer.
- Score 2 for each C answer.
- Score 3 for each D answer.

Score	What It Means
0–2	Pretty perfect score, but you might want to dial back a teeny bit. So the next time the couch is calling when it is workout time, hit the snooze button.
3–5	You are in a good zone. You are working to stay fit and healthy but not being fanatical about it. Stay the course.
6–8	Not bad, but you could do better. This is a great time, pre-baby, to learn how to better care for yourself.
9–12	Hmmm. How about thinking of this as a bit of a wake-up call? Take your pregnancy as an opportunity to prioritize you and your health habits.

Not Selfish—Self-Nurture

The concept of self-nurture can be difficult to adjust to. While it is often confused with selfish behavior, self-nurture is simply taking the best possible care of yourself (essentially treating yourself the way you care for everyone else). Think of it this way: Being selfish is meeting your own needs at the expense of others. Self-nurturance is about meeting your own needs in harmony with the needs of others.

This topic comes up frequently with my patients. Some of them worry about being selfish while they are pregnant. A part of them wants to attend to feeling hungry or tired as soon as the feeling hits, but they don't want to impose their need for food or rest on those around them. They want to put their feet up at the end of the workday but feel guilty for "giving in" and taking a pass on going out to dinner or seeing a movie or a show. Entertaining may feel beyond you; you don't want to have to look good for visitors or clean up or make food (especially if you are feeling nauseated). On the other hand, if you *love* to entertain and it energizes you and is a welcome distraction, by all means go for it.

The fact is, many women are not all that used to meeting their needs as soon as they arise. We are all used to skipping a meal so we can truly indulge over dinner with friends, so feeling famished is the sacrifice we make. But when you are pregnant, that is not such a good idea. You may be used to pushing yourself and ignoring discomfort, but when you are pregnant, resting and eating when tired or hungry aren't options; they are necessities.

Listening to your body and acting on what it is telling you is not selfish behavior; it is self-nurturing behavior. Self-nurture is a wonderful way to get through pregnancy. It's the best way to support your nutritional needs, get the right amount of exercise and rest, and reduce stress. The physical, spiritual, and practical skills you learn to nurture yourself now can be used again and again throughout your life. Remember, if you don't feel your best (if you are tired or hungry), then it is much easier for anxiety or stress to take over your mood and behavior.

Keep in mind that it may look as if you are only taking care of yourself, but when you are attending to your needs, you are really taking care of your baby. For some, it is relatively easy to be "good" once they are pregnant. Others can chafe at being restricted and feel resentful over the new rules they need to live by because it is hard for them to give up what they are accustomed to. If they are used to eating sushi and they can't have it during pregnancy, then they automatically feel deprived. Frankly, it's hard for anyone to be told no and be given a list of things one cannot do. For women who are already self-restricted (especially about food), they can feel overwhelmed with what they cannot do: OMG, I can't do *all* of this? It's okay to be ticked off at what you can't do—no sushi, no alcohol. It's annoying to be told you cannot eat or do something, or to have to change your favorite Friday lunch with friends from sushi to something else because you are pregnant. Or to sit in the lodge while all your friends are skiing during a weekend ski trip. But keep in mind that you are only limited by these noes for the duration of your pregnancy. I've said it before, but it bears repeating: Pregnancy is time limited. Any changes you have to make now are temporary, because after the baby is born you can go back to eating sushi and schussing down the slopes. It may seem as if there is a lot to give up, but during pregnancy there are some key areas that you can focus on, make some adjustments to, and not feel deprived.

Changing what you eat and drink, especially during holidays or other celebrations, is challenging. It can be difficult not to drink alcohol at social events if that is what you are used to. It's hard because you feel as if you are missing out on the fun, but it's also hard because you realize how stupid people can get when they are drinking and you have to suffer through it stone-cold sober. Somehow, along with being pregnant, you may find yourself repeatedly anointed as the designated driver. If you can, bring along a pregnant friend to social functions. Or seek out the other pregnant woman in the room. There is something to be said for having someone to commiserate with when your office party this year is being held at the local Sushi & Sake.

For many of my patients, alcohol is one of the trickiest areas to navigate. Not drinking alcohol is usually the first "tell" that someone is pregnant. I had a patient who was trying to get pregnant and had not yet conceived. She hosted a holiday party where three women friends (all of whom would ordinarily have had a social glass of wine or two) passed on having a drink. The hostess knew immediately they were all pregnant even if they weren't saying so. They hadn't wanted to tell her because they knew she was in the midst of trying and had not yet conceived. Although she was happy for them, she was so sad at the way she found out.

A newly pregnant patient of mine was trying to figure out what to do because she wasn't ready to tell, but a particularly nosy friend was coming for a party. My patient knew if her friend saw her drinking soda, everyone would know about her pregnancy before the end of the party. So I recommended that she buy a bottle of nonalcoholic wine and keep it hidden in her kitchen. That way she could sip away and her friend would stay in the dark.

Another woman, who wasn't yet ready to tell her extended family that she was pregnant, was faced with a dilemma at a family gathering. Her brother-in-law served her up her favorite vodka martini complete with olives and onions. She snuck into the kitchen, dumped the alcohol, and refilled her glass with water—complete with the olives and onions. She said it tasted about as awful as you would expect.

It can be uncomfortable to be in a social situation where people are drinking and be the only one who isn't. It's okay to feel resentful, but keep in mind that you are not drinking for a very good reason. Be sensible on behalf of your baby. No alcohol, no drugs, no smoking.

Food for Thought

If you are like most women, you have spent some time (or all of the time!) in your life on a diet or restricting your eating in some way. When you are pregnant, you need to let go a little. Pregnancy is not license to throw eating carefully out the window, but you do have different nutritional needs when you are pregnant. I'm not a nutritionist, so if you are confused about what to eat and in what quantities, consult with a nutrition expert or talk it over with your OB. The basics are not terribly difficult: You should be eating healthful food. Healthful means the good stuff like fruits and vegetables, lean meats, calcium-rich foods, and whole grains (but take it easy on the processed carbs). You'll have to give up sushi, unpasteurized cheeses, and deli meats for nine months, but you can do it. There are studies that suggest this is the safest course to take. I also recommend staying clear of artificial sweeteners. There is nothing definitive about them one way or another, but in the absence of any long-term studies I'd say better to err on the side of avoiding them where possible.

As I tell my patients, if there is any potential for later regret, don't do it. Don't make yourself crazy, but you don't want to be beating yourself up later for something that you ate or drank while you were pregnant. If there is some issue with your baby, you don't want to be wondering if it was the piece of yellowtail that you had at lunch that time. In all likelihood, that solo piece of sushi won't be the culprit, but why take the chance? Again, talk with your OB or nurse-midwife about nutrition during your pregnancy. She will be monitoring your weight gain at your appointments, so it's a perfect time to bring up any questions you have about diet and nutrition. You can also check out the Web site for the American Congress of Obstetricians and Gynecologists for its recommendations.[1]

Your OB will definitely let you know about the foods you should eat and those you should avoid. He or she will also probably give you some guidelines on portions.

If you had been taking prenatal vitamins before you conceived, talk with your doctor about any vitamins you should continue with now that you are pregnant. If you hadn't been taking them, talk to your doctor or nurse-midwife about getting a prescription right away. Some women feel nauseated when they take prenatal vitamins, so if they bother you, take them at night before you go to bed.

Eating for Whom?

When it comes to determining what to eat, I tell my patients that it is better to focus on what you *can* eat. It's much less stressful and anxiety producing. Besides, have you ever noticed that when you think about what you can't do, it's all that you want to do? If you struggle with this, it might be beneficial to make a "yes" list of the foods you can eat. Obviously, the foods to avoid won't be on there (so you can put them out of your mind), and you'll have a long list of options to eat at any meal as well as to snack on. You can even add desserts! Many of my patients are surprised when I say "Yes!" to dessert.

Once, when I was at a conference, I ran into one of my patients who had stopped at the dessert table. She looked both relieved and guilty when she saw me. She told me she was struggling with whether to have fruit or a brownie for her dessert (and she really loved brownies, but she was pregnant and didn't want to do anything to damage her baby). I told her to go ahead and eat the brownie. She was six weeks pregnant, and the baby was the size of a grain of rice. One brownie wasn't going to hurt. I went on to tell her, and I'm telling you, that your body is programmed to meet the nutritional needs of the baby before it kicks in to serving your needs. So, know that if you are sensible and follow the dietary guidelines that your OB gives you, you will be okay. Notice that I said "sensible." Having a small brownie for dessert is okay; having a pan of brownies as your meal is not.

When some women feel anxious or stressed, they reach for comfort foods, and while they may feel marginally better in the moment, they often regret the overindulgence later, leading to more stress and anxiety about what their eating has done to their bodies and their babies. Moderation is key, but if you overindulge on occasion, it's not cause for panic or major concern. Unless you are being monitored for gestational diabetes or another condition that requires dietary restrictions, sitting down with a bowl of mac and cheese or some Ben & Jerry's may actually be just what you need. Foods that are high in carbohydrates make up most of the common comfort foods. This is not something I recommend that you do on a daily basis, but it can be a nice treat once in a while.

The human body is forgiving and resilient and is protective of the fetus. However, we just don't know the thresholds: Will one piece of sashimi cause a problem, or does it take twenty-five? So the best course of action is to not beat yourself up for any perceived transgression and go with the accumulated wisdom about the foods and activities that are recommended during pregnancy. Avoid anything that is questionable because it is better to be cautious. In most cases, there is wiggle room. The only exception is listeria. There is no room for error, so the CDC recommends avoiding raw sprouts, raw milk (unpasteurized), soft cheeses, deli meats and hot dogs (cold, not heated), and smoked seafood.[2]

Exercise

Exercise has a positive effect on mood. And studies indicate that physical exercise can protect the brain from stress-induced depression.[3]

In fact, exercise is as effective in treating mild to moderate depressive symptoms as are most antidepressant medications. Exercising when you are pregnant can benefit both you and your baby. Studies have indicated that the more fit you are, the shorter your labor will be and the easier it will be to get back into shape after the baby is born. This doesn't mean that you should go out and obsessively exercise in order to try to have a short labor. It doesn't work that way. But it doesn't mean that you should discontinue your current exercise activities either. The general rule of thumb is that if you were doing the exercise before you became pregnant, you can do it while pregnant. There are a few exceptions— skiing, parachuting, and horseback riding—because the risk of injury to yourself or to your baby is so great. Common sense should come into play here: If it seems risky or if there is a chance of falling, pass. The rule of thumb for pregnancy is if you are in doubt, don't do it. Always ask your doctor or nurse-midwife for guidelines.

And if you haven't done much in the way of exercising, now might be a good time to start. Begin with something gentle, like walking or prenatal yoga. If you are taking a class or working with a trainer, be sure to let the instructor know that you are pregnant. He or she can make modifications for you. Toward the end of your pregnancy, you may not feel up to your usual routine, so you can always take the intensity level down a notch. Walk less far or reduce the speed of your usual walk. Reduce the incline on the treadmill and lessen your pace.

Another option for keeping exercise in your life is to take a class that is specifically geared to pregnant women—yoga, water aerobics, a fitness class. There will be accommodations that make allowances for your belly, adjust for the change in your center of gravity, and protect your joints (your ligaments naturally loosen as you progress in your pregnancy). Taking a prenatal yoga class can help you to engage your mind along with your body. Many women report that yoga gives them an opportunity to reduce stress through the meditative aspects of the practice.

Another advantage of taking a prenatal class is that you have the opportunity to meet other pregnant women. The social aspects of exercise are great, and making the connection to someone who is at the same stage in pregnancy as you are can be wonderful. You may not only find a new friend but gain a new perspective on how to cope with any issues you are facing.

Walking is an excellent exercise for when you are pregnant (and even when you are not). Slipping on a comfortable pair of sneakers will be welcome to your feet. You can plan some walking routes in your neighborhood or around your workplace if you want to take a break during lunch hour. Having a planned route near home can come in handy, because you can continue your walking routine later with your baby in a baby sling/carrier, stroller, or jog stroller. It will be great for you both to get out of the house, and if you have a familiar route to take, it will be that much easier to lace up your sneakers and go. In addition to the movement, getting some fresh air and additional vitamin D from the sunshine are bonuses from a brisk walk. Walking is also something that you can do with a friend so you can have some company as you exercise.

Holly is twenty-four weeks pregnant and has always been active. She worked out four or five times a week before getting pregnant, usually with running as a part of her routine. Now she doesn't have the desire to run and has slowed down to taking long walks. She has said that when she is feeling anxious, "exercise is a great release." She has also found companionship is beneficial. "I walk with a friend who is a couple of weeks ahead of me in pregnancy, and it is nice to be with her."

Ask your OB for recommendations, ask the trainers at your gym or local Y, ask friends if they have taken classes that they enjoyed.

Toward the end of your pregnancy, you may be uncomfortable and find it difficult to move. Don't beat yourself up if you can't exercise the way you would like to, because your inactivity is temporary. If you can't move the way you'd like, you can try something simple like breathing exercises or arm exercises.

Sleep

Many women spend a lot of time worrying about diet and exercise, but few pay attention to sleep—except to complain that they are not getting enough. The truth is, sleeping well is rare at all stages of pregnancy. However, it is important for your mental and physical health to pay attention to sleep and learn how to get the amount of sleep you need. There is no set number of hours you need to get while pregnant; it's very individual, and it might be significantly different from before you got pregnant. Use your body as a guide. If you are yawning all day and feeling drowsy most of the time, you need to get more hours of shut-eye. If you wake up before your alarm and feel relatively alert most of the day, you might have found the right number of hours for you.

Sleep is fast becoming an intensively researched subject,

and it turns out that sleep has an incredible effect on everything from mood to weight loss. Sleep is huge. Some studies have shown that how much sleep you get while pregnant can have an effect on your mood, it may be related to your risk of having a premature birth, and it may be related to your risk of developing postpartum depression.

If you are not sleeping well, you will not be at your best. Sleep is a time when your body recharges its batteries, your immune system does its routine maintenance, and your hormones regulate themselves to keep your body's systems running effectively. Without sleep, you can be grumpy, hungry, tired, unfocused, and generally not feeling, thinking, or operating as well as you should. Pregnant women should focus on sleep as much as they focus on nutrition. And maybe even more!

Don't assume you have to suffer with sleep deprivation just because you are pregnant. Suffering can bring on anxiety; suffering and no sleep can make you more emotional, less focused, and feeling out of sorts.

Why Can't You Sleep?

There are some common physical reasons that will interrupt your slumber: You need to pee, your back or leg muscles hurt, or you have heartburn. It's important to figure out the triggers for waking you up or keeping you up so you can troubleshoot for them prior to going to bed.

If getting up to pee is the problem, take a close look at what, and how much, you drink after 6:00 p.m. While fluids are important during pregnancy, too much can interfere with sleep. If you are drinking liquids because your mouth is dry, try sucking on a mint or hard candy. Something to assess is whether or not you really have to pee. When most people wake up in the middle of the night, they automatically trudge to the bathroom, whether they really need to pee or not. If you wake up, take a minute to check in with your body to see if you really need to pee or if you can settle yourself back into sleep.

If you struggle with heartburn, you can try sleeping in a more upright position, propped up with pillows or a bed rest pillow that has a back and arms. Have chewable antacids on your bedside table so you can take something quickly to ease your symptoms. Try to keep track of the foods that end up giving you heartburn, and avoid them as much as possible (you'll only be taking a break from the food for a little while and can eat it again once the baby is born). Also, try not to eat anything immediately before going to bed.

When you have muscle aches or pains, there are a number of things you can do. Have your partner give you a back or leg massage. A warm hot-water bottle on the affected area can also bring relief. For leg aches or pains, put a pillow between your legs. Experiment with different sleeping positions. One side may be more comfortable than the other. Use pillows to support your back or legs.

A number of women have told me that they used all sorts of pillows to help them find a comfortable sleep position. Some used all the bed pillows they had, and others bought pillows that are specifically designed for pregnant women. The only downside to the pillow invasion is that your partner might feel a little crowded out. When Fran was pregnant with her twins, she said, "I used a Snoogle—a body pillow. I swear by it; my husband, not so much!"

If worry is keeping you up (and that midnight imp can be wild: What if my baby has two heads? What if I don't love my baby? What if my baby doesn't love me?), try the cognitive restructuring approaches discussed in chapter 4 (see also appendix I). Remember, it's perfectly normal to worry when you are pregnant, but if you let your worry run away with you, you will not sleep, and lack of sleep will only make you more anxious.

Before trying any herbal or over-the-counter medications to help you sleep, please consult with your OB or nurse-midwife. Just because it worked for your co-worker's cousin doesn't mean you should go ahead and do it. Because there are no true safety regulations on herbs, you need to be especially careful about taking them. Also, over-the-counter and other sleep medications can be habit-forming, so you want to exercise caution when taking anything. So, unless your OB says otherwise, avoid over-the-counter sleep aids. Sometimes the home remedies are the best: Stick with a glass of warm milk or some soothing chicken soup.

Some techniques you can use to get your sleep schedule on track are the following:

- Try to go to bed at the same time each night and wake up at the same time each morning, even on weekends.
- Even if you are tired, limit the length of time you nap during the day because it can interfere with your ability to fall asleep at night.
- Don't watch TV or use a laptop, tablet, or phone immediately before going to bed. The light from these devices interferes with your sleep cycle.
- Do some gentle stretches before bed, but refrain from strenuous exercise.
- Practice meditation or do some relaxation techniques (see appendix I).
- Listen to gentle music.
- Use a white-noise machine.
- If something is troubling you, write it down in your journal before going to bed, and then you can attend to it in the morning.

Spirituality

Taking care of your physical needs can help keep your stress low and anxiety at bay, but many women find that exploring their spiritual side helps them find some peace of mind while pregnant. If they have not been active members of a house of worship, many women and their partners make the decision to return to some form of spirituality so they can raise their baby with a traditional faith. Some feel that returning to the worship of their childhood feels like coming home. Others look to a different spiritual tradition from their childhood experience. Try a variety of experiences; I have a pregnant patient who went with her husband each week to a different church. She said that finding the right congregation was important to her because it will become her child's place of worship. After about six weeks of church shopping, they found the perfect fit. They felt embraced by the community, liked the minister, and are looking forward to the christening of their baby there.

Nurturing You

Let's face it, taking care of your unborn baby is priority 1, 2, 3 (sorry partners/spouses!), but you need to put your needs on par with those of the baby. Taking some time for yourself is an excellent way to find a bit of peace and relaxation, reduce your stress, and do something that makes you feel good. Diana has had three children, and none of her pregnancies were the same. She has experienced preeclampsia, developed a skin condition that caused intense itching of her belly, and worried with each pregnancy about something different. She found solace in listening to music and visiting with her family, but she also said, "Retail therapy and chocolate work too!"

Physically, there are many things you can try. Go ahead and get a pedicure (who cares if you can't see your toes; the experience will allow you to take a break from the day, have your feet taken care of, and relax for a bit). If you've always wanted to have a facial, go out and get one. Besides, your skin may behave differently during pregnancy, so having a new cosmetic routine can be a welcome change. See if your local spa has a pregnancy massage or other services for pregnant women. Going to a salon or a spa may seem self-indulgent, and it is, but it's okay to take some time for yourself to give your mood or energy a boost. Also, taking some time to feel good about your appearance isn't only about the cosmetic aspect. It can give you a break in your routine and a boost to your mood. If money is tight, invite some friends over, especially pregnant ones, and paint each other's toes.

Meeting a Stranger in the Mirror

Some patients tell me that they see their reflections in mirrors and don't recognize themselves; this can be especially jarring if you catch your reflection in a mirror or window when walking down the sidewalk. One woman said, "Looking in the mirror and not enjoying what I am looking at triggers negative feelings." Keep in mind that everyone looks different when she is pregnant. Your face will be fuller; there is more fluid in your body because your blood volume has increased in order to support your baby.

When you feel as if you are seeing a stranger in the mirror, here's something you can tell yourself:

> *I may not like the way I look now, but it's the way I need to be in order to nourish my baby.*

Honestly, most people aren't looking at your face; they are looking at your belly. Everyone expects women to look different when they are pregnant; it's part of pregnancy. But these changes don't mean you can't try a new hairstyle, change up your jewelry, or wear all black. Whatever makes you feel better—go for it!

You Don't Have to Suffer—You Can Make Yourself Feel Better

Being prepared can reduce anxiety. When you are faced with a pregnancy-induced issue, come up with a strategy that will work for you, and put the plan in place. Make a list of issues, their triggers, and the antidotes. By putting yourself back in the driver's seat, you are taking control of the situation. Action can help keep anxiety at bay.

If you are suffering from sciatica (back pain that shoots

down a leg), figure out what sitting or standing positions are most comfortable so you can move to them immediately once you feel the pain. Bring a pillow for your chair or a footstool to your office.

Many women find that the smell and taste of citrus can counter the feelings of indigestion and nausea. So carry some lemon drops with you. Use lemon-scented soap or hand lotion. Find a citrus toothpaste. Ginger has also been known to relieve nausea.

In Your Bag or at Your Bedside

Here are a few things you might consider having handy so you can give yourself the care you need:

- water
- saltines
- lemon or citrus hard candies
- peppermints
- ginger candies
- antacid
- tissues

Come up with strategies that can help you feel better. Create a cozy routine for when you get home at night. Put on comfortable, loose clothing, put your feet up, get a foot massage or soak your feet in warm water, ask for a back rub, use some citrus-scented lotion for your hands, sip a cup of fruit-based herbal tea, have your favorite meal ready for heating (or have the take-out menus ready for ordering in). It will give you something to look forward to at the end of the day. You can also think about little things you can do for yourself throughout the day. Take an herbal tea break. Take a stretching break. Take a walk. Read a book. Anything that gives you a chance to relax and regroup is great.

When you are pregnant, you really want to be comforted (I want my mommy!), so if your mother is not available, you'll need to do for yourself what she might do for you. A cozy robe, slippers, and your favorite soup can be welcome respites at the end of the day. Be gentle with your spouse and mother-in-law; they may try to "mother" you, which may rub you the wrong way. Remember, they are trying to help you, so watch for creating conflict with your partner and mother-in-law over these issues. Remember to be clear about what you need but also to be polite if their attentions or efforts to help you aren't welcome.

⤸

Strategies for Self-Care

The things that make you feel better may not work for another woman, so it's worth finding out for yourself what helps you relax, turn down the negative chatter in your brain, and find some space for yourself and your baby. Here are some things that have worked for other women:

- take a walk
- take a shower
- exercise
- talk to my husband
- talk to my mom
- talk to my best friend
- listen to music
- get out of the house
- meditate
- read
- watch my favorite movie

Keeping Guilt at Bay

A lot of what we "know" can be harmful is more of a correlation between an action and the result. If you smoke, you are *more likely* to get lung cancer; if you drink, you are *more likely* to have cognitive or liver problems. Pregnant women who drink alcohol frequently are *more likely* to have a child with fetal alcohol syndrome. But remember that this doesn't mean that there will be a major issue if you are around secondhand smoke or if you had a glass of wine before you knew you were pregnant. Unfortunately, current research hasn't answered the question of how much is safe. Most women who smoke and drink during pregnancy have had healthy babies. But the risk is there, so it is better to be safe than sorry.

We really live in a control-freak society, and many

people think that if they do *x*, *y*, and *z*, they will be guaranteed a particular result. The truth is, you cannot do it all, but you can avoid the extremes in eating and exercising, and you can use common sense in all that you do. Plus, you have the support and advice of your doctor or nurse-midwife; don't forget to use that resource. The bottom line is to control what you can. This applies to what you eat, drink, and think. Finding ways to take care of yourself physically and mentally can bring peace of mind. You will feel better because you are taking charge of the situation and minimizing the risks. That is really the best you can do. In fact, the best you can do is almost always more than enough.

Chapter 6

Belly Support

In a world where people post, tweet, and Instagram nearly every thought, meal, and life event, we can get used to feeling as if everyone were interested in everything we are doing. In fact, there are probably many people (some you would expect and some not) who are interested in your pregnancy—your partner, your parents, your partner's parents, the lady at Costco (more on her later). You will find that people are excited for you and there are those who want to share your experience. It may also be surprising to find that some of the people who you thought would be interested seem less excited, supportive, or involved than you thought they would be.

Anna is surprised about her husband's lack of support. "Because it's an easy pregnancy and I've been active and not emotional, he almost forgets that I'm pregnant. He doesn't step in and do things for me or pick up the slack."

Brittany says, "I assumed my mom would be more involved. I'm the youngest, and I thought she'd be there like she was for my brother and sister."

There are people, including yourself, who may have pre-conceived (so to speak!) notions and expectations about your pregnancy and what it will be like. With the wealth of knowledge that can come from family and friends, you may feel as if you have amazing resources available to you. And you do. Keep in mind, however, when it comes to preg-nancy, generally people do not present balanced views. Their expectations about pregnancy are at either end of the spectrum—either all good (glowing!) or all horror stories (morning, noon, and night sickness!). This is not to say that you won't have balanced information from your OB or other medical professionals or that your childhood friend will tell it like it is without freaking you out. It's just that people tend to go for the dramatic when talking about pregnancy and how you will be feeling. Dramatic stories are newswor-thy and can be entertaining. A routine pregnancy isn't.

Frankly, it's really not up to others to tell you how to feel. How you feel is up to you, and no matter what you will not be wrong. Your pregnancy is your pregnancy. No two pregnancies are alike. Even identical twins won't have identical pregnancy experiences. That being said, it is only natural to look to your family to see if you can scope out what your pregnancy experience might be like. Most women, logically, ask their mothers about their pregnancy and birth experiences. There is, in fact, a possible genetic link to morning sickness, so if your mom was sick when she was pregnant, you might be too. But much depends on the circumstances. If your mom was miserable, nauseated, and tired when she was pregnant, she might have told you many stories about her experiences, and you may expect the same for yourself. Before you start preparing for 24/7 morning sickness, check into her circumstances. Did she drink or smoke, was she on her feet all day, did Dad expect meat and potatoes on the table the minute he came home from work? Was she looking after other children and didn't have time for herself?

The things that might have contributed to your mom's feeling badly may not be in your life. Maybe your father didn't help around the house, but your partner does. If this is your first child, you won't have to contend with caring for another child as well. There are many different circumstances, and even if you don't feel well, your individual situation and how you react to it can alter how much it affects your life and your mood.

The reverse can also be true. Mom might have had it easy because she was able to rest during the day and didn't have to be on her feet for her job, have long hours, do shift work, or have a long commute to work. You may be juggling your pregnancy with your job and other obligations, and that can be a drain on your emotional and physical resources. Yes, there is a genetic relationship, *but* that doesn't mean it is inevitable that your pregnancy will mimic your mother's.

My mom told me that she had been sick 24/7 when pregnant with me, so I sort of expected that for myself. I was surprised when my morning sickness went away at the end of each of my first trimesters. I think she was jealous!

Conversely, one of my most delightful patients was told by her mom that she hadn't had a second of discomfort during her own pregnancy. So my patient went into her pregnancy expecting to feel marvelous, scheduled all sorts of work trips and dinner parties, and then spent the first fourteen weeks of her pregnancy vomiting on a daily basis. So you can never know. One study actually showed that women who are pregnant with a girl tend to have more nausea and vomiting. But some of my sickest patients have had boys. Go figure.

The crazy thing about pregnancy is that your second pregnancy may be completely different from your first! Carole spoke about the differences between her first pregnancy and her second. She is now the mom of a toddler and a newborn. "During the first pregnancy, I was *happy* expecting, but I had a rough delivery and a colicky baby. In my second pregnancy, I wasn't so happy. I was depressed, and the closer I got to my due date, the depression symptoms increased. I thought about taking medication but talked about it and decided not to. It was terrifying because of my experiences with my first (no depression). My mood was so *off*. I couldn't sleep. I couldn't rest. I had a lack of interest in things. I was incredibly irritable. It was hard and exhausting not to give in to being grumpy and irritable."

While Carole's example shows extreme differences between pregnancies, it just drives home the fact that no two pregnancies are alike, and rather than being focused on how others are doing, or have done, with their pregnancies, you should keep in mind that your pregnancy is unique to you.

Many people do not like feeling out of control, and this can be so true during pregnancy. Try to focus on what you can control, such as eating foods that don't trigger heartburn, napping when you have the chance, going for a walk when feeling draggy, calling your mom or a friend when feeling lonely, watching funny reruns on TV, or listening to your favorite music when you need a lift.

Expectations

You probably have some expectations for what you will hear from other moms, sisters, cousins, and friends. You may be expecting nurturing and support, and you will hopefully get that; just don't be surprised if some of the information you hear is negative. Because no two pregnancies are alike, you are very likely to hear conflicting information from friends, family, and others. You may hear some over-the-top stories because a normal pregnancy or delivery is not headline-worthy or very dramatic. (Of course it is exciting for you and gets top billing in your life, as it should.) But because the negative stories seem to rise to the top, it's easy to expect the worst.

This is especially true when you start to think about labor and delivery. When you have no prior experience and don't know what to expect, it can be scary. The only deliveries you might have seen were in movies, and they are played to great dramatic or comedic effect (so not terribly realistic) or on a medical crisis show where everything possible could go wrong (also not terribly realistic). You can really start to worry about how you will feel and about what will happen when your baby is born. Tess said that the hardest thing for her about being pregnant was the fear she had about delivery. She says, "I was terrified of labor and either me or the baby ending up with some horrible physical problem. I heard terrible stories and was so worried about what would happen." All turned out well, and both mom and baby are completely healthy.

It is safe to assume that your pregnancy is a blank slate and you will do whatever you can to treat your physical and emotional symptoms. You will use the resources available to you and do what's right for the baby. The first line of defense when it comes to any questions about your pregnancy or any worries you may have is to speak to your OB, nurse-midwife, or other health-care provider. His or her depth of experience can be a great source of information and comfort for you. Keep in mind, however, that OBs hear women complain all day, so they may not raise an eyebrow over common issues that you bring up.

So that you don't get overwhelmed with information from others (the friend who sends you the latest article on diet, the co-worker who wants to tell you the story of her cousin's traumatic birth experience), you need to take a stand. You need to be clear about how much input you want from other people. The watchwords here are that it is *your pregnancy*, *your body*, and *your baby*! (Yes, it is your partner's baby too, but you will be the primary recipient of a wealth of unsolicited advice, attention, and others' expectations.) If you set limits now, you will be well practiced at it when it comes time to set limits with others about any input you want regarding your baby and how you are parenting/raising her. I frequently advise my patients to put it out there early in the pregnancy. Be clear that you do not want to hear horror stories of any sort. And in terms of unsolicited advice, a noncommittal "hmmm" might well discourage the average person from continuing to pepper you with information and advice. Other, non-average souls might need a bit more of a direct approach. I am talking being assertive here, not aggressive. I do believe that most people mean well, but people's need for attention and tendency for exaggeration can take over in these situations.

You may find conflict closer to home. Friction about the baby may arise between your parents and your partner's parents. It may be surprising to see them in disagreement if they were perfectly civil and cooperative with each other for your wedding. The thing is, with weddings there are generally accepted rules to follow, but with a pregnant daughter-in-law there are no specific guidelines on the role the parents play. Conversely, there might have been many unhappy "discussions" between them regarding your wedding, and yet they somehow have a united front over their new grandchild. At least for now!

Be aware that your mother-in-law is the one most likely to feel left out. She may get a chip on her shoulder if you share information only with your mom about how the pregnancy is progressing. One of my patients, Margaret, has a lovely close relationship with her mother but is completely intolerant of her mother-in-law, Anne. I obviously have not seen Anne in action but have, in fact, heard a number of stories that attest to her bossiness and lack of consideration. However, Margaret refused to share any information about her pregnancy with Anne, which led to many frantic phone calls, texts, and e-mails asking what was going on. This began to negatively affect Margaret's relationship with her husband, because he felt caught between the two women he loves. I understood that Margaret didn't feel inclined to share her joy with someone she really didn't like or respect, but I could also understand how helpless and shut out Anne felt. Margaret and I had several conversations about how she could include Anne more in her pregnancy and life, in the least painful ways possible, such as e-mailing Anne ultrasounds or asking for input on specific things such as high chair recommendations. This led to a lot less drama, and in fact when Margaret's baby arrived, Anne calmed down and was actually helpful with her new grandchild.

Carole has a unique approach to sharing information with her mom and her mother-in-law. She has a good relationship with both women but says that her mom and her mother-in-law have very different approaches. "My mom will say, 'Deal with it' or 'Here's what you do'; she is very much about making a plan. My mother-in-law will tell me to 'cry it out' and ride my emotions to the end. So I go to either one for what I'm most needing at the moment. Both are supportive and helpful."

A lot of people care about you and your baby, and they will put expectations on you and your pregnancy based on their own experiences. You may have certain expectations about pregnancy that you have picked up from culture, media, family, and friends. So that you can get the support you need throughout your pregnancy, it's helpful to take a look at expectations and see what you can do to keep them realistic and manageable.

Managing Your Expectations of Others

The best way to manage your expectations of others is to figure out what you need. Do not expect anyone to read your mind. Be aware that what you need today may be different from what you need tomorrow. You might want to inhale a cheeseburger on Tuesday, and on Wednesday the mere thought of it can make you feel queasy. You may want your mom to come to your ultrasound, or you may want only your partner. You may not want to have the usual Sunday brunch with the in-laws. Tell those around you. Nicely. Particularly your partner. Your partner wants to help, but he's probably not sure what to do. Without being a prima donna and overly bossy, you can *ask* for what you want. You co-created the baby, but it's your body growing it, and it may still feel unreal to him. Be sympathetic if he isn't thinking "baby" 24/7. Men don't spend all day thinking about the baby and may not want or need to talk about it all the time either. It's not because your partner doesn't care; it's because his body (and mind and emotions) haven't changed. He is the same. You, on the other hand, are changing in ways that are both visible and invisible. It doesn't mean he's not excited or on board with the new baby that is coming. It's just that his life hasn't shifted to being baby-centric the way yours has. Also, because he isn't thinking about the baby all the time, he may not realize that you need help with things you would ordinarily do yourself. He can't anticipate what you want. You need to tell him. This is the time for you and your partner to come together as a team so that he can help you but also so that he can help you with others.

I see this all the time when I do couples counseling. The wife feels ignored and declares that he is a selfish lout, and he looks bewildered and says that he has no idea how to make her happy. You need to become aware of what your needs are and express them in a healthy way. He has no idea that his eating a slice of anchovy pizza in front of you is the most revolting thing you have ever witnessed and triggers your gag reflex. Brittany said, "My husband couldn't even *talk* about red meat. I couldn't even *hear* about it!" So Brittany let him know that it bothered her, and he refrained from any talk of steak or other meat in her presence. He also completely took over the food shopping when walking into a grocery store made her sick to her stomach.

Another one of my patients was furious because her husband didn't buy the fresh fruit she wanted. Seriously. I suggested that she tell him exactly what she needed when he went food shopping, and she realized that in fact her eating had changed considerably since she got pregnant (in a good way; she was making a big effort to eat more fruits and vegetables and less junk food). The issue was that she hadn't told him. So he continued to buy the meat and potatoes (and chips and ice cream) that they had always eaten. And he was completely bewildered when she blew up at him when he brought the groceries home. Here he thought he was being such a good guy, doing all the grocery shopping so his pregnant wife could rest on the sofa, and he gets home and his wife flips out that he didn't buy strawberries.

You also have to pay close attention to how you are asking or telling those around you what you want. Swift mood swings are so common during pregnancy that you might not be fully aware of how you are behaving. You may think you are being rational, but you may not be. Try to be reasonable. You need to stand up for yourself, but you need to be fair. If you feel nauseated and you can't cook, don't! But let him know so he can order in something or can cook something for himself while at the same time getting something for you that you can and will eat.

Sometimes, particularly around food, you can feel like a two-year-old. You want it, and you want it *now*! You can go from being completely uninterested in food one minute to being ravenous the next. There is something to be said for keeping a granola bar or small snack with you to take the edge off your hunger and so you won't be so sharp with whoever is with you when your hunger hits. I personally recommend keeping a small buffet of snacks in your desk, your purse, and your car.

Pregnancy isn't an excuse to try to make everyone around you wait on you hand and foot. Don't forget that you can do things for yourself even if you are pregnant. Exceptions exist of course. If you are on bed rest for any reason, you should follow your doctor's orders and not be up making food or doing housework and so on. Do what you can and ask for help with what you can't.

Quiz
Where Is Your Support?

1. **How are you and your partner coping as a couple?**

   a. *It has clearly brought us closer together.*
   b. *He likes hearing about the baby; sometimes he seems jealous of the attention I am getting.*
   c. *He wants to know about problems but isn't interested in day-to-day.*
   d. *I feel that he's not emotionally invested in the pregnancy at all.*

2. **Are you satisfied with support you are getting from your family?**

   a. *Despite some shopping rivalry, both sets of grandparents give me/us the support I/we need.*

b. *Mom and I are having a good time sharing the pregnancy; my mother-in-law has been a bit intrusive.*

c. *Parents don't seem all that interested, but the in-laws are providing some support.*

d. *All the parents are busy with their own lives and not particularly attentive to my pregnancy.*

3. How supportive are friends?

a. *They're super excited and planning a shower.*

b. *Friends with kids are involved; single friends don't seem to get it.*

c. *A few friends have been there during the pregnancy, but I feel isolated from other friends.*

d. *All my friends are single or going through infertility, so I don't have anyone to talk to.*

4. How comfortable are you being pregnant on the job?

a. *My boss is so excited for me that I'll have to ban him from the delivery room.*

b. *My boss and colleagues are professional but not supportive.*

c. *Colleagues have acknowledged that I'm pregnant, but I don't feel free discussing it at work.*

d. *I feel that my boss is looking for a way to fire me so he doesn't have to support me during my maternity leave.*

Scoring: Give yourself the following points for each answer you circled, then use the chart that follows to determine how stressed you are about being pregnant:

- Score 0 for each A answer.
- Score 1 for each B answer.
- Score 2 for each C answer.
- Score 3 for each D answer.

Score	What It Means
0–4	You seem well cocooned and supported. Cherish your connections.
5–8	It sounds as if you are doing well in terms of people in your life. It might take a bit of work to keep it up after the baby comes.
9–12	I assume you feel somewhat lonely and unsupported. Make your needs known to people who have the capability to support you.
13–16	You are likely feeling alone. Talk to people you trust and work to make more connections. Try a pregnancy yoga class or a support group; seek out members of your church. Look for pregnant high school friends on Facebook to share your experiences with. Consider seeing a therapist either alone or with your partner.

Your Partner

The best way to assess your partner's expectations is to ask him how he's doing. Ask him what he wants to do during the pregnancy. Does he want to be at every doctor appointment? Does he want to talk to the baby? Come with you to classes? Read any books? Will he tour the hospital with you? Will he take Lamaze or other childbirth classes?

As mentioned previously, the baby is an abstract concept for him. Even if he has seen a sonogram that shows the baby has the same-shaped feet as he does, it's still not completely concrete for him. However, his level of awareness and involvement can change dramatically once he feels the baby kick. His reaction may surprise you. He may react very emotionally. Physically, it's all about you. Emotionally, it's all about both of you. He may react differently than you do, and that's okay. You might be all thoughts of baby names, adorable outfits, and stroller brands, and he might be lying awake at night worrying about college tuition. Many men handle marriage more easily than the responsibility of parenthood. In my experience with the men I counsel, a man's relationship with his father can have a big effect on how he feels about becoming a father. Remember also that you might well have had far more experience with and exposure to babies than he has. Many men are terrified of small babies!

Some men bring their own worries to the situation based

on their experiences in their families. Carole's husband has a difficult relationship with his younger brother, and when they were having a second child, he worried that his kids would have the same struggles. He was also worried that he wouldn't love the second baby. She says it all worked out fine: "The moment our second child was born, he was crying and fell in love."

You may also have to let him know specifically how you feel. He may not get it. He might not understand the extent of how ill you feel. He's thrown up, but he's never been this sick before. There is a huge difference between a hangover (which is temporary and self-induced) and pregnancy nausea. In pregnancy, you could be feeling this way for days or weeks. Talk to him about it when you are feeling somewhat better, and explain what you need him to do for you if he is there when you are throwing up. Think about what you need and communicate that to him. Make a list. *This is what I need when I am feeling nauseated: no cooking in the house, no coffeemaking in the house, no talk of food, food commercials muted on TV, a cold washcloth/ice chips/saltines/mouthwash.* You get the idea. If he has no idea how you are feeling, he has no clue how to help you.

Just to show you how no two pregnancies are alike (even for the same woman), I had a patient who was severely sick during her first pregnancy and dreaded being pregnant again. But the second pregnancy was great. You just never know.

The Moms

There aren't many guidelines on how mom and mother-in-law should behave toward each other or toward you while you are pregnant. How these relationships shake out is heavily influenced by the relationship you had with them before you got pregnant. Depending on your relationship with your mother-in-law, she may consider herself to be your other mom, and you may be very close. If so, she may expect you to come to her with any problems or questions, but at a time when you can be emotional and vulnerable, it is very natural for you to seek comfort from the mom who raised you. If you are feeling sad or anxious, your mom may already know the exactly right thing to say. Your mother-in-law may feel slighted or left out. Try to think about your mother-in-law's feelings. It's her grandchild too. Don't exclude her from the pregnancy or shopping for the layette. But, based on your relationship with her, you might need to set limits.

When I was pregnant, I continued to talk more to my mom than to my mother-in-law, but I was sure to share information with them both. We made a conscious effort to keep my in-laws posted on any developments, but it wasn't on a daily basis. I could be more direct and frank with my mom. I could say, "I feel fat; can you go and buy me some yoga pants?" With my mother-in-law, I kept her in the information loop, and if she asked if she could do something, I'd accept her offer and encourage her.

Some in-laws are not terribly interested in your pregnancy, which can be a little sad, but they will hopefully be excited about the baby. Pregnancy becomes the center of your life, and that may not be the case for everyone. Try not to judge. Maybe your mother-in-law is a private person and doesn't want to intrude. Maybe she is trying to be respectful of you and your privacy and is waiting to be asked to be involved. The number of grandchildren already in the picture can make a huge difference as well. If your parents already have six grandchildren and this is the first for your husband's parents, it shouldn't be shocking that they show far more excitement. And vice versa. One of my patients actually became far closer to her mother-in-law because of this. Her own mom had a posse of grandchildren and didn't show nearly as much ecstasy about the newest grandchild as the mother-in-law did. My patient had many fun shopping expeditions with the new grandma-to-be.

Many of my patients who are very close to their mothers don't feel moved to share with their mothers-in-law, which causes some conflict with their partners. I try to persuade them to share something with the mothers-in-law but to do it on their own terms. Some ideas are to send her a PDF of the sonogram and take her along shopping. Find some way to include her, and in doing so, you will set the tone for when the baby is born. If you are super picky about something like a stroller or a car seat, then ask for her input on something else. Don't set her up for failure by asking her to buy something that you had already hoped to buy yourself.

Another patient of mine had preemie twins, and while she was still in the hospital, she asked her mother-in-law to buy some clothes for the babies. The mother-in-law was thrilled to have something helpful to do, and it took one thing off the new mom's list. In-laws can also come in handy if you have little ones and are expecting. You need more help the second time around, and babysitting can be a wonderful gift—for Grandma and Grandpa as well as your little one.

⚘

It's All in a Name

Family members often have expectations about what you will name your baby. My advice on this one is that at the very least, until you have chosen a name, don't announce your contenders. People will feel free to tell you what they think of the name or that there was someone who had that name in their second-grade class and they hated that person. Family members may expect you to continue a family naming tradition. It never ceases to amaze me how intrusive people are about names. They seem ready to comment, criticize, and get involved when your baby's name is none of their business. The only two people who should decide on a name are you and your partner. You can make it clear that you are not accepting suggestions or input. Pick a name that you and your partner both love.

Another tactic is to not tell anyone the name until after the baby is born. People are less likely to criticize a name if there is a baby involved. If you present the name as final and attached to your baby, then people are less likely to weigh in with any negative comments on the new baby's name.

That said, if you name the baby after someone on one side of the family, it may cause hurt feelings on the other side. If there is any way you can balance it, such as first name from one side and middle name from the other side, it might be worth the effort. If there are no nice names and you can't see giving your baby a middle name like Ralph, consider using another name that starts with the same first letter and let the person know that you have chosen the name in his or her honor.

Your Boss

At some point, you need to tell your boss that you are pregnant. The right time will vary depending on your workplace and your relationship with your boss or manager. If there are any work-related responsibilities that could pose a risk to your baby, you may need to reveal your pregnancy earlier than you are comfortable with. But in general, tell him or her at a point where you are comfortable sharing the news, because it will get around to your co-workers. Before the conversation, be sure to check your company's policy regarding maternity leave. If you don't have paid leave, try to save your vacation and sick days. Many companies don't give paid leave, so let your boss know that you will be using your available vacation days and sick days once the baby is born. Work with your boss about your maternity leave (who will cover your workload, whether you'll be in touch throughout your leave, and so on) as well as a plan for your return.

You should also be familiar with the Family and Medical Leave Act,[1] which, depending on the size of your company, guarantees you up to twelve weeks of unpaid leave with job security. Also check and see if you are covered by short- or long-term disability, which can provide a chunk of your salary for six to eight weeks.

Your boss may be happy for you as a person but also concerned about you as an employee. Your boss's responsibility is the well-being of the department or the company, and she has to think about the big picture. She will be concerned about how your pregnancy will affect your work performance and if you will come back after your maternity leave. She will expect you to continue to do your job and contribute to the company throughout your pregnancy and to make a plan to come back after your maternity leave.

You can expect that depending on the type of work you do, your boss will grant you accommodations for your job (perhaps you can't stand for long hours or lift a certain amount of weight). It would be a good idea to find out what your company's policies are along with any state or federal regulations. You should know that you can't be fired for being pregnant, and if you need to be off your feet while working, talk to your boss, talk to HR, or call your state government so that you have all the information at hand should an issue arise with your employer. Ask your OB if you should have any accommodations and get a signed note to document what you need. If you work with food and you are nauseated, perhaps there is another task you can take on, or maybe there is another shift you can take when you are less unwell.

Other company policies you should look into are short- and long-term disability insurance, which might cover you if you have medical issues during your pregnancy. Your partner should check his employer's paternity leave policy. Think about using his leave creatively. If your mom is coming to stay with you for the first week that you and the baby are home from the hospital, have your partner take the second week off so you'll have two consecutive weeks with someone at home with you. Knowing the company policies and having a plan in place can take some of the pressure off when you are sorting out how you will work through your pregnancy.

Work responsibilities can be a source of anxiety. Anna found that her mind was racing about getting her work done before maternity leave. She recently got a new boss, and it's not a great situation, so she's not particularly happy at work. She's considering switching jobs, but at thirty-two weeks the timing isn't great. She assumes she will still be at the same job when the baby is born, so she signed her child up for the day care at her current place of employment. She knows if she changes jobs, she'll need to take on the added worry of finding day care for her baby.

So she has three things on her mind at a time when work should not be the thing she is most worried about. Try not to make any work-related decisions hastily. I don't mean to sound insulting, but emotions do tend to run higher during pregnancy, making a situation seem more dire than it may be in reality. Try to talk through worries, decisions, and perceived obstacles with other people to in effect bounce your perceptions off them. I remember lying awake at night, freaking out about work, and when I mentioned my obsessions to my husband or a co-worker, even I had to admit that I was, perhaps, exaggerating the problem. A good way to get a fresh look at a problem is to write about it. Literally take pen to paper, and write down your thoughts and feelings about the issue. Not only is it cathartic, but in all likelihood the solution will become clear.

Your Friends

By and large, your friends should be thrilled for you when they hear you are pregnant. Depending on where they are in their lives, they may have differing expectations for their relationship with you now that you are expecting. You may find that the single friend you met weekly for after-work drinks has found another friend to hang out with. Or, you may have a single friend who is so excited about your pregnancy that she starts planning a shower the minute you tell her that you are having a baby. Friends who are pregnant at the same time as you may be a great source of comfort (Let's take a walk together and compare notes) or competition (You only threw up twice? I threw up five times—on my boss!). Friends who have children may not see your pregnancy in quite the same light as you do. From their perspective, it's something they've been through, and it isn't as big a deal, because they are excited about the phase of life they are in now. To them, pregnancy can seem routine despite how new and exciting it is to you. One of my patients recently announced a much-desired second pregnancy, eight years after the birth of her first child. A good friend actually reacted to the news by asking my patient if she really wanted a baby at this point in her life.

Connecting with women who are pregnant and, ideally,

due around the same time as you can launch some wonderful new friendships or rekindle old ones. It's fun to hang with people with whom you have things in common. But be sure that you like the person as a friend, not just because she is due the same week as you. It's also possible that you may forge a bond in a prenatal class and then, once your babies are born, find you don't feel drawn to spend as much time together. This may be especially true if one of you has a really easy baby and the other has a more "sensitive" one.

Be mindful when talking about your pregnancy to friends who are not pregnant or who don't have kids. You may not even be aware of friends who have been trying longer than you and not succeeding. Most people who go through infertility don't tell anyone, even their mothers. So your friends who are childless, or have an older only child, may well be suffering in silence. Be aware that your pregnancy may be an enormous source of pain for them. They don't hate you or your baby, but it is too difficult for them to hear about your pregnancy. Take their lead on how much contact they want to have with you. It may be none at all, and please don't take it personally. Invite them to your baby shower, but don't pressure them to attend if they show any hesitation. Once their infertility is resolved through treatment, adoption, or acceptance, they will, hopefully, come back into your life. Many women struggling have the hardest time with pregnancy and babies but are more comfortable with older children. Let them come around in their own time. Continue to include them in your life, but don't press them to attend any baby-centered events.

Getting the Support You Need

The best way to get what you need is to first think about what you need. It's rare that any of us takes the time to stop and think, "What do I need?" You need to think about things like *what makes me feel better; what makes me feel worse.* Many pregnant women think the only option they have is to *endure* their pregnancy. You can do better than that. Recognize your needs and see who in your life can meet them. Partner? Other family members? Co-worker? Friend? Church? Self? (Remember, you need to care for yourself too.)

Pregnancy prepares you for having a baby, and you want to be in good physical shape for the marathon that is newborn life. In the first year of life, a baby develops more than it will in the rest of its life combined. You will be busy, and getting some practice asking for help now will benefit you (and your baby) in the future.

Labor and Delivery

Delivery is one of the most joyous experiences, but it is very intimate—both physically and psychologically. For the first-time mother, labor and delivery can be an anxiety-producing prospect. If you are having your first child, you really don't know how you will react physically and emotionally. The big question that will come up is, who will be in the delivery room with you when your child is born? The bottom line is there are two people who should be expected to be with you—your partner and your doctor (and eventually your baby!). Anyone else who attends your labor and delivery is up to you.

Some women choose not to have their partner in the room. Maybe that will be the best choice for you and your partner. Maybe he faints at the sight of needles or blood. Maybe he's not great in a crisis and would wind you up instead of calming you down. Have a frank conversation (or two) with him about his comfort level. But don't leave the conversation or the decision until you are on the way to the hospital when you are in labor. Have it when you can both discuss your expectations and concerns. The two of you, together, need to decide what is best for you both.

Many of my patients have wanted their mothers with them as they labor and deliver. There really isn't any reason she shouldn't be there, but you'll want to be sure your partner is okay with having your mom in the delivery room. I have already told both of my daughters that I would really, really love to be with them in the delivery room. Seriously. Given that the older one just started college, I am guessing (hoping) they have lots of time before they have to decide.

If other people say they want to be in the delivery room, you can thank them for the offer but say you only want your partner or whomever it is you *do* want there. Addie had a friend who asked if she could be at the delivery. It wasn't even one of her closest friends and was, in fact, a relatively new friend. As Addie put it, "I am very private and modest about my body. I am the woman in the locker room who *always* has a towel on and who practically gets changed *in* the locker, so the idea of having anyone other than my husband at the delivery was, to my mind, completely off the charts! I gently declined and let her know she'd be the first one to know if I changed my mind."

Labor and delivery is all about what *you* want, not what others expect for themselves and what they want. I have had many conversations with husbands about why their wives need to be in charge of who is in the delivery room. To be honest, I tell them that if there is ever an occasion where they plan to push a seven-pound package down a far smaller canal, they can invite anyone they please to watch. That usually does the trick.

I am a firm believer in having a plan in place, but, especially with a first child, you need to be willing to veer from the plan if, in the situation, it doesn't feel right. Circumstances may change, and you may rethink your carefully thought-out birthing manifesto. That's okay, as long as your OB or nurse-midwife is okay with any adjustments and your health and the health of the baby are not put at risk.

Things often feel different one moment than they did the moment before. My sister, brother-in-law, and I never talked about my being in the delivery room when their baby was born. My sister called when she went into labor; I drove up from New York to Boston in the middle of the night, popped into the labor room to say hi, and by mutual consent never left. You really won't know how you are going to feel until it is happening. Which also means that if/when you invite others to be there for the birth, they have to know that you have the right to change your mind at any time. Designate your partner, in advance, to be the one to ask them to exit (when you ask him to take care of it); you don't want to get into a discussion about it while you are in labor.

Birthing Options

There are many options available for who will guide you through your labor and delivery. It can be an OB or a nurse-midwife, and you can hire a doula (a trained labor- and delivery-support person). Doulas are a great option for having someone assist you in preparing for giving birth and helping you throughout the process. If your partner is nervous about being your "coach" or isn't able to assist you, you can get a doula or a labor coach. They are not cost prohibitive. Or, if you have a friend who has skills (nurse-midwife, doctor), he or she can be your backup labor coach. In my experience, labor and delivery nurses, because of their training and wealth of experience, can be amazing sources of support, information, empathy, and creative ideas. But be aware that when you are in labor, the labor and delivery nurses are going to come and go. You might absolutely love the nurse assigned to you when you arrive, but a few hours later, when you are about to need to push, she is going to leave when her shift ends.

You also have options about where you will give birth. Some women want to give birth at home with their family around them. Personally, I'm nervous about home births. While there is no reason to medicalize labor and delivery, the stakes are too high to have a baby without easy access to services should something go wrong. If your family expects you to have a hospital delivery, hear them out. A nurse-midwife or a doula can be an excellent option for a hospital-based birth with personalized support if you think you want more than what your local hospital already offers.

At the end of the day, it is your delivery. If you are young and healthy, there is a 95 percent chance of a delightful delivery at home. Just be sure you are informed of the risks and have a contingency plan if something should go wrong.

If the medicalization of delivery makes you nervous (or if the thoughts of delivery trigger your anxiety), take a tour of the delivery and maternity ward of the hospital where you plan to have your baby. In many hospitals, the labor and delivery rooms are set up to be quite homey and less institutional. Obstetrics is a big business, and the hospital where a woman gives birth is where she will most likely seek future medical care for herself and her family. It's in the hospital's best interest to make labor and delivery as positive an experience as possible. Again, pregnancy is not a medical condition or an illness. If you are young and healthy, there are few risks, but there are some. Being in a space that can provide medical attention for yourself or your baby, if needed, is a safe backup.

So make a plan, but be ready to change it. And don't be reluctant to change even if it's just because you feel like it. You can't know in advance what will happen, what you will want, or how you will feel, so you have to go with what is going on in the moment. It is not a failure to change your plans. There is no harm in having a backup plan in place if things don't go the way you expect. I always talk to my patients about epidural anesthesia, even if they are completely committed to natural childbirth. Having a plan B and even a plan C in the back of your mind is always good insurance.

Self-Advocacy

It's rare to stop and think about what makes us feel good; we tend to focus on what makes us feel worse. But in order to get what you most need, it is helpful if you can focus on what makes you feel better. During pregnancy, you need to keep an open mind about what you want or need because changes can come on a daily basis. You will undoubtedly need the support of someone throughout your pregnancy. However, in getting that support, don't turn into a diva. Pregnancy doesn't mean you get to sit on the couch watching reality programs or binge watching your favorite TV show and snapping your fingers for your next glass of water. Don't be bossy. But if you are vomiting, you really should get a pass on making Thanksgiving dinner for twenty-eight. The only sure way to get a pass is to ask for it. Check in with what you are capable of, and don't push yourself beyond your limits. Avoid using pregnancy as an excuse to get out of things just because you don't want to do them. Skipping making dinner or other household chores once in a while is okay, but taking a hiatus from everything for nine months is not.

Be clear about your needs, and be sure that the person you are asking *can* meet that need. Remember there is a big difference between can't and won't. You can do a lot for yourself, but don't be shy about asking your network of family and friends, because hopefully they will do their best to give you all the support you need. Be aware that your emotional needs are just as important as the physical ones. If you are feeling anxious or depressed, that is just as compelling as being exhausted or having heartburn. The key is to check in with yourself about how you are feeling and learn whom to contact for support. The list of potential people can include not only your partner and family but a therapist, clergy member, or your OB's nurse.

Chapter 7

Talking Your Way Through Pregnancy

I WAS TALKING to a reporter recently who was doing a story on couples' issues with the age-old question: Is it better to try to resolve a fight before you go to bed or to wait until the morning? I told the reporter that the healthiest relationships are based on trust, honesty, and good communication. This is never as important as when you become parents together, so pregnancy is an ideal time to either polish your communication skills or learn new ones.

In general, the best way to get your needs met is to practice healthy, effective, authentic communication. Communicating well during your pregnancy will facilitate any conversations you have about your pregnancy with your partner, health-care provider, friends, co-workers, and family. Good communication skills can also prevent conflict and misunderstandings and help to repair any rifts that may occur. Good couple communication is the creator of healthy relationships, while poor communication leads to unhealthy relationships.

Nothing will change a relationship more than having a baby. The arrival of that bundle of joy transforms you into *parents*. And that transformation is nothing short of amazing! It's a wonderful and exciting time for both of you. But it also represents a massive change in your lives. Those nine months waiting for your bundle of joy are a great time for you, as a couple, to develop into a family and a great opportunity to work on communicating with each other; it's not just plenty of time to find the perfect crib. And learning to communicate well with each other will come in handy when the two of you are trying to put together that perfect crib.

To be a healthy family, you first need to be healthy communicators as a couple. If you are going to have a baby with your partner, you need to be able to talk to your partner. Pregnancy is a dress rehearsal for parenthood, so if you are struggling with communication now, then it will be far more challenging when you are parents. If you are really struggling with communicating with your partner, it would be a good idea to go to a couples' counselor to establish healthy communication skills before you have the baby.

Communicating Changes

As you transition into your role as parents, changes happen for both of you. But for you, the changes are primarily physical, and as we've discussed, those physical changes have an effect on your mind and mood. Not feeling great makes most people more irritable, and the person you love the most, your partner and the parent of your child, may be on the receiving end of a lot of that irritability.

Honestly, I didn't know it was possible to feel as awful as I felt when I had morning sickness (that lasted throughout the day). I remember trying to explain to my husband what it felt like to be nauseated 24/7, but until you have experienced it, perhaps words cannot describe it. I am intrigued by the new Chinese effort to show men what labor feels like; they put electrodes on the abdomen of the expectant dad and shock him enough to mimic contractions. I assume these men are far, far more empathic during labor. But as tempting as it may be, it would probably not be ethical to give men nausea-inducing medication for weeks at a time!

If you are having tough physical symptoms, you do need to give yourself a bit of a break; it's difficult to be civil when you are suffering. My old boss got pregnant when I was in my mid-twenties, and she was the first pregnant person I knew well enough to ask what it was really like. Her answer: "Have you ever seen the movie *Alien*?"

However, just because you are pregnant doesn't mean you have to be rude. When you catch yourself snapping, instead of writing it off as pregnancy hormones, simply say, "I'm sorry." It will only take two seconds of your time and can go a long way to keeping the lines of communication open. Recognize your mood swings. Do everything you can to try to get as much sleep as possible, because lack of sleep affects mood. Be aware of when you are not being delightful or delighted and act accordingly. When you recognize and apologize, you mend your relationship and keep the conversation going.

Another aspect of honest communication is giving your partner insight into what you are feeling. If you constantly write off your behavior as hormones running amok, he won't have a sense of when you might need some extra TLC or need to call your doctor or mother or therapist. Also, if you are always at DEFCON 10, it's difficult for him to respond appropriately.

When I first worked with chronic-pain patients, if I asked them about their pain level, many of them would report that it was a 10 on a scale of 1 to 10 all the time. But if you had them keep a pain diary, it often showed that it was a 4 while watching TV and a 6 during dinner. The same thing goes for pregnancy. You might believe that you are tired and irritable and have heartburn or nausea all the time. But I assume there are times when you actually feel a bit better. Let your partner know. He may feel guilty that you are suffering so much, so if/when you have a good moment, let him in on it. It will be good for you as well to note when you feel okay so that you don't have (or give) the perception that your pregnancy is awful all the time. It is human nature to focus on our own suffering, and we tend not to notice when we feel fine. When you have a cold, all you notice is how hard it is to breathe and how annoying it is to have your nose run all the time. But when you are healthy, you don't stop and think, "Wow, I feel great. My breathing is so clear, and my nose feels terrific."

Try to understand things from your partner's perspective. He might feel resentful that you can't do all the things you used to enjoy doing together. He may be upset that you aren't taking care of him the way you did before. One of my pregnant patients told me that her husband had complained to her that she wasn't giving him back rubs anymore. That felt completely irrational and annoying to her, because she was the one with back pain from the pregnancy, but she missed the message he was sending. Yes, it is irrational and somewhat selfish that he still wanted back rubs from a woman who hadn't seen her toes in weeks, but I suspect he was trying to say that he missed her doting on him. My recommendation? Take turns with the back rubs.

Some men are nervous about being affectionate with their partners when they are pregnant for fear of hurting them or doing something to harm the baby. One woman thought her partner would think she was so sexy when pregnant. It did not seem to be the case, and she began to think he would be happier if she was quickly back to her "normal" self. When they spoke about it, he said he was anxious about having a healthy baby and saw her pregnancy as something to get through; he couldn't wait until the pregnancy was over and the baby was safe and sound. It wasn't so much that he didn't find her attractive as that his worries for their baby affected how he was viewing her.

Another couple I saw weren't being intimate at all, and it bothered both of them. But when I asked them why, it was obvious they had never talked about it. When questioned, she said she didn't want to be naked in front of him because she felt so huge and unattractive. He said that his wife had never been so sexy, he loved seeing her pregnant, and he was hurt that she was shunning his advances. Once each of them knew what the other was thinking and talked it through, they got back on track. It is amazing what a little conversation can achieve.

You may feel upset that your partner isn't taking care of you the way you want him to and at the same time feel frustrated that you can't do it all now that you are pregnant. Don't take it out on him or those around you. When we feel bad and lash out at others, we are usually making the completely illogical assumption that they can read our minds and should know exactly what to do to help us or make us feel better. The trick is to rise above the quick reaction and take some time before you speak or respond. Ideally, you want your partner to be honest, considerate, and empathic, so you should extend the same courtesy to him. Think about what you need, think about what your partner needs, and figure out ways to work on meeting each other's needs while at the same time not forgetting to nurture yourself.

Quiz

In Terms of My Relationships with Those Around Me . . .

❧

1. **When I need something from my partner . . .**

   a. *I freely ask whenever, whatever, however, and he's happy to oblige.*

   b. *I feel guilty that I can't hold up my end, but he hasn't complained.*

   c. *I notice that when I ask for things, he stomps around more than usual.*

   d. *He says that pregnancy is not a disease and I should get off my butt and take care of myself.*

2. **When a family member announces that she is going to move in with you for a month after the baby is born, you . . .**

   a. *Thank her for the offer of support but say you and your partner haven't yet figured out how much help you need. You tell her that you'll let her know as soon as you've reached a decision.*

b. Say, *"Thanks, we'll get back to you. We've had a lot of offers, and we need to think about them."*

c. Say, *"We have things worked out, but if we need you, we'll call."*

d. Say, *"There is no way we'd have you with us for a month!"*

3. **What will you say if your boss asks you, point-blank, what you plan to do about work after the baby is born?**

a. *"My current plan is to come back to work full-time. If anything changes in that plan, I will let you know."*

b. *"I haven't begun to think about that, but I'm pretty sure I'll come back to work."*

c. *"I'm not sure if it is even legal to ask the question." And then stomp off.*

d. *You know you don't plan to come back, but you want to cash in on maternity leave, so you plan to tell him the day before your leave ends that you are not coming back. In the meantime, you say that you are.*

4. **When you are sick and tired of friends telling you what they did, giving you advice, how will you handle it?**

a. *Listen sweetly when they tell you what they did and thank them for their input. Then you'll do what you think is best.*

b. *Thank them for the input, and let them know that you will be handling this pregnancy and bringing up the baby slightly differently than they did theirs.*

c. *Immediately put your hands over your ears and tell them you are not seeking any input; you'll do it your own way.*

d. *Tell them, "I think it is pretty ironic that you are giving advice, considering the circumstances of how well your pregnancy, labor, and delivery went."*

5. **When strangers offer unsolicited advice, opinions, or observations about your belly, your appearance, and so on, you will . . .**

a. *Smile and say, "Thank you for your helpful advice."*

b. *Say, "We've got this covered."*

c. *Say, "We've made it a policy not to take advice from people we don't know."*

d. *Say, "Who are you to be giving me advice? Do you really think I'd take advice from a stranger about something as important as my pregnancy and my baby?"*

Scoring: Give yourself the following points for each answer you circled, then use the chart that follows to determine how stressed you are about being pregnant:

- Score 0 for each A answer.
- Score 1 for each B answer.

- Score 2 for each C answer.
- Score 3 for each D answer.

Score	What It Means
0–4	You have terrific communication skills and are doing a good job getting your needs met.
5–9	You are adept at getting your needs met but might want to slightly tweak your tone.
10–14	There is a good chance that you mean well but you aren't communicating that message. Maybe practice a few responses?
15–20	Ouch. I assume you feel overwhelmed and it shows up as irritability toward others. Try taking a deep breath before responding. Think about how your responses are perceived.

Say What You Mean, Mean What You Say

You and your partner are both probably excited, scared, and ambivalent, but your emotions might not be in perfect sync. You may be excited just when he is feeling ambivalent—and vice versa. In this mix of emotions and expectations, you need to be very careful about how you communicate. Speaking reactively will not help either of you to get what you want or need. There will be times when you just can't do it yourself.

You may feel too woozy to drive; you may be nervous about the ultrasound and need support and companionship.

In the heat of the moment, it's easy to lash out, but it's best to avoid name-calling, accusations, and labeling. For example, when he starts frying the fish he just caught and the smell is making you insane, you should not simply say, "You're a jerk!" and run out of the house. You need to more fully explain what you are thinking and feeling so that you can open up a dialogue.

The basic formula for couples' communication is this:

It makes me feel _____ when you _____

because _____.

For example: It makes me feel **so frustrated** when you **do things that trigger my nausea,** because **it makes me feel that you don't believe how sick I am really feeling.**

♣

You are at a party, and by 9:00 p.m. you are so tired that you literally can't keep your eyes open; but when you tell him you want to leave, he rolls his eyes and asks if you can just hang on for another hour because he is having such a great time. You should not call him inconsiderate, storm off, and drive yourself home, leaving him without transportation.

You should say, "It makes me feel so uncared for when you disregard how tired I am because it makes me feel that you don't care how I am feeling and that your friends are more important to you than I am."

Your partner can't truly understand what you are going through, particularly physically. You can tell him that you are tired or nauseated and feel terrible, but to him (especially at the beginning of pregnancy) you *look* the same. Your partner has to learn to trust that when you say you are too tired to do yard work that you truly are and that what you say about how you feel is accurate. You also need to be honest about how you feel and not use your pregnancy as a "get out of _____ free card." It's not fair to do otherwise. It's also not fair to assume that your partner will just "know" how to help you when you feel unwell, stressed, or down. You need to communicate without accusing ("You never . . .") or expecting him to read your mind (saying "Oh, nothing . . ." while thinking to yourself, "You should know what I need without my having to ask!").

You might feel as if lying on the couch reading books about pregnancy is all you want to do, but he feels fine and wants to do the same things you've always done together. He may also be eager to do all the things you won't be able to do when you have an infant. You can find a way to compromise. Maybe you are super tired during the week and don't feel up to going out for dinner. Tell him, but at the same time make a plan for going to your favorite restaurant over the weekend when you may be less wrung out. He'll also have to bend a little and take into consideration the limitations put on you due to your being pregnant. A weekend of downhill skiing followed by the all-you-can-eat sushi bar isn't going to cut it. But if you are used to doing outdoor activities together, take a nature walk or ask your OB if it would be okay for you to cross-country ski or snowshoe and find a place to eat that you can both enjoy.

On the other hand, you may need to take some time to see things from his perspective. He may be a little freaked out by the changes your body is going through. Physically, he won't be personally affected by the pregnancy, but many partners feel a huge sense of responsibility for their future child. They also worry about what having a baby will do to your relationship. That worry doesn't mean he wants the baby any less, but he is probably aware that for the foreseeable future what he wants and needs will tend to fall behind what the baby wants and needs. Tell him not to worry; in eighteen years or so, he'll get to the top of the list again.

Stages of Communication

The way you maintain good communication throughout your pregnancy doesn't change much from trimester to trimester.

What changes are the issues that come up and how they need to be addressed. Again, the watchwords for good communication are "honest," "considerate," and "empathic."

You may feel needier in the first and third trimesters. It's likely that you will be more uncomfortable and will need to ask for more support and comfort. By the second trimester, you are more visibly pregnant, but most women feel better and sometimes have a bit more energy. That's often when the proverbial "nesting instinct" sets in.

Some women find it difficult to ask for and accept help. If you have always been self-sufficient, it can be very hard to ask to be cared for. Pregnancy is not a disease or a disability, but it has an effect on what you can and can't do. So it's okay to ask for help when you need it. Keep in mind that you are really asking for help for the two of you; you are not being selfish, but you are looking out for your baby.

It can feel as if the equal partnership you have in your relationship shifts if you need more now or can't do the things you are used to doing. Frankly, that balance will shift throughout your relationship and may experience significant changes once the baby is born. For now, you have an important job to do, and you may need some extra help to get it done. The tasks that you typically take care of and those your partner takes care of may need to be reassigned. If you are nauseated and are usually the one to do the grocery shopping, ask him, ask your mom, ask a friend, or order groceries online. If you ask your partner to do the shopping, you can take on something that he usually does, like doing the dishes. The trick is to ask for help only when you really need it; don't burn him out, and don't overdo it with friends or family. Hundreds of years ago, women helped one another, but we generally don't live in communities like that anymore. It's up to you to ask for what you most need from those who you know can give it to you.

Sometimes you may find yourself in a position where you can't easily ask for help. It can be hard to work during the first trimester because you may be tired and nauseated but haven't reached the point of telling anyone at work yet. Your partner can be a sympathetic ear as you find your way through this time period.

Critical Communication

One of the most crucial communication points in your pregnancy is labor and delivery. Labor and delivery is a very intense time, and it's a good idea to talk about it before you rush off to the hospital. It would be helpful to have a conversation with your partner regarding your expectations of his role during the birth. With a first child, it can be difficult to know what you will want because you have never been in the situation before. Even if you don't know precisely what you want, in my opinion you get more say here than anyone else. Once the baby is born, your partner has equal rights, but when it comes to labor and delivery, his job is to say, "Yes, dear." Your job is to let him know that you'll do your best to tell him what you want. Even if you don't know what you want yet.

At the end of the day, it's your body, so what you say goes. If you want to wear a particular pair of polka-dot socks, to watch Olympic wrestling, to listen to Gregorian chants, or whatever, as long as it's okay with your health-care team, you should be able to do so. You need to be as comfortable as possible to do the hardest work of your life. Of course any decisions regarding the baby's health should be made equally between you and your partner. And if there are any safety issues to consider, as can arise with a home birth, you need to have a discussion about them—preferably before a problem comes up.

Partner's Role During Delivery

- Support her
- Coach her
- Encourage her
- Pamper her
- Breathe with her

Be flexible and roll with what she needs (a back rub may feel great one minute and not the next, so don't take it personally if she tells you to stop)

Communicate for her when she needs it with the OB, nurses, or other hospital staff

You may want someone else in the delivery room with you, apart from your partner. This could be your mom, a doula, or a friend. If you do want someone else with you, it will help your partner to be as supportive as possible if you talk this through with him. For many women, it's not that they don't trust their partners to do the right thing in the delivery room; it's just that they are more comfortable having some female support—particularly from women who have already had children.

Frankly, having men in the delivery room is a fairly recent development; it hasn't always been that way. You have to know your partner and talk to him. Some men get queasy in medical situations. He won't be of any assistance if he doesn't feel his best. It's a great idea to talk to each other about your expectations and fears. Many couples attend birthing classes together to better understand the process and for the partner to learn what can be done to support a woman during delivery. That can be a great time to talk about what you want during delivery. Going out for a meal or coffee after the class can provide the perfect opportunity to talk about these issues when they are fresh in both of your minds.

One of the most common issues I see in my practice is that the woman wants her mom there but not her mother-in-law. This causes tension with her partner, because he worries that his mom will feel left out. As I said previously, my general rule of thumb is that what she wants in the delivery room, she gets. But please take your partner's thoughts and wishes into account. Maybe compromise; your mom can be with you for labor but not delivery. Or his mom has visiting privileges when you are not contracting, but she can't come into the delivery room. Or do what one of my patients did: not tell his mom that she was in labor until she was pushing!

Liz says that her in-laws are a source of anxiety. "The in-laws want to be at the hospital when I deliver; this makes me anxious. I will not have them in the delivery room. I have a plan, and I just want me and my husband in there. They didn't ask; they just assumed that they should come. There is a baby in there that is their grandchild, but I don't know how my body will react or how tired I'll be. I had concerns, so I called the doctor, and he talked to my husband about how to handle the situation."

The takeaway message here is to talk openly about both of your expectations, desires, and fears regarding labor and delivery. You made the baby together, so both of you should have some say in the baby's exit strategy. But in the case of a tie, choice goes to the mom-to-be.

How to Communicate What You Want

If you feel that your needs are unmet, the first thing to do is to think about what you *really* need. This can be more challenging than you think because your needs can change minute by minute, hour by hour, day by day. What you desperately needed yesterday, you may find you don't need today! A chocolate chip muffin was the go-to thing that made you feel great on Monday, but by Wednesday you can't stand chocolate chip muffins and want a banana. Let your partner know. If he brings you a muffin, yelling at him because he thought he was doing something nice for you isn't fair. It also doesn't help if you take the muffin and don't let him know, gently, that you are tired of eating muffins or that they give you heartburn. If you don't say anything, he won't know how best to help you, and his well-intended gesture can begin to annoy you.

You also don't want to turn into a pregnancy diva. The way to avoid this is to keep in mind that it's not what you ask for but how you ask. I've had patients who seem to expect the world to revolve around them when they are pregnant, and they make the people around them miserable. If the people in your life have the capacity to help you, then ask them for help, but do so nicely. Think about what you ask for. Is it reasonable? If it's unreasonable, then ask with humor.

When pregnant with my first daughter, I had a craving for corn dogs. The craving hit at 11:00 p.m.—on a Sunday night. My husband sighed as he put his coat on over his pajamas, ready to go on a corn-dog hunt, and the sight made me laugh so hard that I lied and told him my craving had passed. He was relieved when my craving during my second pregnancy was for onion rings and that it only seemed to occur during business hours.

How to Talk to . . .

Your Partner

It's important to say specifically what you need. Don't blame, or he could become defensive. As far as he is concerned, you are the one who has turned into an alien. Living with someone whose moods, body, cravings, and sleep habits can shift minute to minute can't be easy.

> **Don't say:** *"I know it's my turn to make dinner, but I'm not doing it. I can't. I'm pregnant. You need to do it for a change."*
> **Do say:** "I am so tired I can't cook; can you please take care of dinner tonight?"

> **Don't say:** *"I am exhausted, and the thought of walking the dog makes me sick. For once, you have to get off your butt and do it."*

Do say: "I'm too tired to walk the dog; would you mind doing it?"

Don't say: *"Your mother is calling and texting me constantly. Get her off my back."*
Do say: "I think your mom is feeling a bit left out of this pregnancy. Can you make a mental note to call or e-mail her several times a week with updates?"

Your Family

In the last ten years, I have observed a change in how the parents of a pregnant woman react both to the pregnancy and to the arrival of the grandchild. Some prospective grandparents are *not* changing their lives when the baby comes. I have seen a lot of my patients get very disappointed at the discrepancy between how they anticipated their parents would respond and how their parents behaved. Grandparents are happy but are *not* overly involved; they are excited but don't go out of their way to help. They come to see the baby and bring a gift but don't make dinner or do the laundry. One of my patients complained that when her in-laws would come over weekly to see the baby, they would literally just sit and hold the baby. They never brought a pizza, took out the vacuum, or offered to help with a meal. They expected to be cooked for and fed. They ended up adding to her workload rather than lightening it.

Alison, now the mother of a toddler and a three-month-old, says that when her mother-in-law came to visit after their first baby was born, "she helped with the baby, but didn't cook or do other chores. We lived near New York City at that time, and my mother-in-law wanted to sightsee. And she wanted my husband to come with her. She was here for the baby and the Empire State Building but not for me! I was so upset that I was left alone. When I talked to my husband, at first he was upset that I was upset, but we talked it out and it was okay."

You might be annoyed with your family if they are not as involved as you expect them to be. Trying to figure out during your pregnancy what roles your parents and in-laws plan to have can help you to avoid disappointment. One of my patients was stunned when her parents made plans to go on an extended vacation two weeks after her due date. But as disappointing as it was, it did give her warning that her parents did not plan to change their lives as much as she would have liked.

On the other hand, some grandparents are thrilled beyond belief and do indeed change everything to be helpful and accommodating. Some cross the line and don't allow the new parents any time alone with their newborn. The key to finding the right balance between too much attention and not enough is, of course, communication. If your parents or in-laws are being awesome, tell them. And if they are being too hands-on, be gracious but clear about needing time alone to bond as a family of three.

Another piece of the family puzzle that can interfere with communication and expectations is siblings. I've seen it often: Sibling rivalry never dies! Much here depends on your family of origin and your ongoing relationship with your siblings. But it can be helpful for you to be aware of certain situations that can stir trouble. Siblings might not be supportive or excited, because they are envious or because they have kids already and don't think it's a big deal. If pregnancy was a breeze for your sister, she might not be very sympathetic to your troubles, because she can't relate. (She might always have thought you exaggerated in the first place.) Siblings might be going through infertility or married to someone who doesn't want kids even if they do. So don't assume your siblings are going to always be excited and helpful. Their issues or challenges might be unknown to you but painful for them.

Louisa, thirty-one years old and twenty-five weeks pregnant, has a younger brother who always gives her a hard time. She said, "When I was telling my little brother about my back pain, he said, 'You know how old you are to be having children?' I couldn't believe he was saying I was too old to be having a baby! By the way, he is only eleven months younger than me, so who is he to call me old? When I told my mom, she said, 'If you want to get your feelings hurt, you know who to call!'"

Margo, who now has a six-month-old, said, "My sister was pregnant with her second child at the same time I was pregnant with my first, and we were in the same week. We spent time together and spoke on the phone. She could be very reassuring about what was coming."

Your Friends

Much about how you communicate and connect with friends while you are pregnant depends on where your friends are in the child process. If a friend is pregnant at the same time, it can be fun to compare notes and give each other support. Or, it can turn competitive. If a friend is going through infertility, it may be understandably hard for her to share your joy. In reality, a part of her is happy for you; it's just that you now have what she wants and is working for and it can be tough to see you get what you want before her. Patients have told me about friends who have disappeared for a time but then were able to celebrate with the patient on their own terms and time. It can be lonely to lose a friend at this time, so it might be helpful to contact her and perhaps connect over the phone and talk about something that is not pregnancy- or baby-centric.

Your In-Laws

I've seen and heard of a range of responses from in-laws. Some who don't get along *do* during pregnancy; some who do get along suddenly *don't* during pregnancy. Pregnancy can cause a shift in the relationship because the in-laws suddenly have a huge vested interest in their daughter-in-law's body; their grandchild is in there!

If your mother-in-law is adding to your stress, put yourself in her shoes. It's hard to be the mother-in-law of a pregnant woman because there is no precedent for this level of her interest in what is going on with your body. Try to include her as much as you can. Remind yourself that your baby is her grandchild as much as your mom's. Sometimes mothers-in-law can be pushy and insecure. But I've also heard stories of mothers-in-law who are wonderful. You need to be fair but maintain the relationship. Be clear about limits and boundaries. If she gives unwelcome advice, say thank you and ignore it. You don't have to be rude or argue; you can simply ignore. Or if she is pushy about something, you can always say a white lie and that you asked your doctor about it and he would consider it.

If you have a good relationship with your in-laws, then keep that going and be the one to update them. If you don't currently have a close relationship, then there is a chance that connection could change over the course of your pregnancy. If your in-laws are triggers for anxiety or you have had problems in the past, you can have your partner be responsible for communicating with his parents. In fact, this might be the best way to be fair about keeping all the parents in the loop.

One woman's pregnancy relationship with her mother-in-law got off on the wrong foot when she and her husband announced, at Thanksgiving dinner, that they were expecting. Before anyone could offer congratulations, the mother-in-law said, "Oh, so that explains the weight gain!" The woman was reluctant to share any information with her mother-in-law after that incident and delegated all updates to her husband.

When Diana and her husband announced that they were pregnant with their third child, her father-in-law said, "Whoops, you did it again! Don't you know how that happens?" She said, "I know he was trying to be funny, but . . ."

Your Boss

Most women tell their bosses they are pregnant when they are comfortable with the world knowing the news. You know your boss best, but it's usually a good idea to approach him when he is not in the middle of a deadline or rushing off to a meeting. It can be a happy or an awkward conversation. The boss might worry about whether you will come back after you have your baby. His job is to keep the company going, and you have to understand his concern about your being pregnant is not necessarily about you as a person but about you as an employee. You might worry about keeping up with the job, and many women feel conflicted about whether or not they will return to work. It can be tough to be an effective employee when pregnant, and it can be stressful to be faced with the decision of whether or not to come back to work, considering all the variables like how to find child care if you do return and what the effect of staying home will have on your career.

Be aware of the big picture at your place of employment, but take time to educate yourself on state and federal laws. Know that you can't be fired for being pregnant; if you need to stay off your feet, then your employer has to accommodate that. Talk to your OB; have a discussion with your boss. Know the law: Family and Medical Leave Act.[1]

It is important to know your rights. A recent case heard in the Supreme Court concerned a woman who said her employer, UPS, did not accommodate her pregnancy.[2]

In another case, a woman sued because, she said, she was fired for taking too many bathroom breaks.[3]

Your Health-Care Provider

The relationship with your OB can be intense. To work most effectively, it needs to be positive and built on good communication. To keep your appointment focused on what concerns you and to keep your doctor apprised of how you are doing, maintain a list of questions so you can stay organized. If something isn't pressing, make a note of it in your phone or tablet and bring your notes to your next appointment. (Ask your partner if he has questions if he isn't able to come to the appointment with you.) The OB's goal is to make sure you stay healthy and have a healthy baby, so he or she is the best resource for any questions you have. I recommend trusting what your physician says over what a friend or your dog sitter might say.

Be aware that when you complain to an OB, it may seem as if he or she is not being empathetic, but it's probably because he or she has seen it all before and is maintaining a professional demeanor. If you say, "I've thrown up ten times today," and your OB doesn't shout, "Oh my God! Poor you!" it's not because he doesn't care. He is listening and constantly sorting what's normal from what is a red flag. *Don't* exaggerate your symptoms. If you threw up three times, say that; don't say thirty even if it felt like that. On the other hand, don't minimize any symptoms, especially anything that appears suddenly or affects your ability to function physically or emotionally. Your health-care provider can't help you unless he or she knows what is truly happening with you. This is especially true about your emotional health. Many pregnant women feel far more comfortable discussing stretch marks and nutritional goals than how they are feeling psychologically. Your health-care team needs to know about the whole package. If you feel fine physically but are anxious or sad, tell them.

Check in with yourself before each visit. Ask yourself to sum up your status since your last visit, in terms of physical symptoms, emotional symptoms, and your overall well-being.

As I mentioned previously, how well you are sleeping can have a huge effect on your health. If you aren't sleeping well, tell your team. They might have some good ideas for you. Do not be embarrassed to talk about being sad or anxious. Many pregnant women have these symptoms, and they are just as important as the physical ones. And they can be just as easy to treat.

Your Therapist

The relationship with your therapist can change when you are pregnant. You may feel less self-focused and more focused on the baby. The concerns or issues that brought you to therapy in the first place might have changed. If you have a male therapist, you might feel disconnected from him over pregnancy issues, but that is okay. Talk it out. If your therapist has no experience working with pregnant women, this may cause some frustration for you. You might be describing how unsettling your Braxton Hicks contractions were during a work event, and if your therapist asks what those are, you might feel as if he doesn't have the skills to support you during your pregnancy. But the fact is, your pregnancy is a temporary condition, and if you are with a beloved therapist who knows you well, it might be worth it to tolerate the pregnancy oblivion and continue to focus on the issues that brought you into therapy in the first place. It is also possible to temporarily seek counseling from someone who has experience in working with pregnant women. I frequently see patients who have their own "regular" therapist but see me for a few sessions to focus on the issues in their lives brought on by their pregnancy.

Strangers

You may find that people are happy to tell you, unsolicited, disturbing stories about pregnancy and give advice constantly. People get weird; it's as if your belly and your baby have suddenly become community property. The same people who would never give you work or relationship advice will suddenly tell you all about pregnancy. Even total strangers! Think carefully how you want to communicate with them. They probably mean well, and assuming that they do, simply being friendly is often the happiest (and easiest) way to go.

Stranger Than Fiction

A few things that women have been told when they are pregnant:

- "In the middle of Costco, a woman pointed at me and said, 'You are having a boy!'"

- "I got constant comments about 'how small' I was and ended up worrying about it rather than being flattered. I was surprised at how unfiltered everyone was about their opinions."

- "People would say, 'Single people usually avoid getting pregnant; why would you do it on purpose?' And they would ask if I wanted a boy or a girl, and when I said, 'A healthy baby,' they thought I was odd."

- "Look at you! You've really popped!"

- "Oh, you'll stay home!"

- "You *must* breast-feed!"

- "Be sure to take the drugs when you deliver!"

- "Another one?! So soon?!"

STRANGER STRATEGY

One thing to do to keep your composure when faced with unwelcome information is to think about the things that people say that make you crazy and come up with a comeback line. It's likely that you will hear the same comment or "advice" from completely different sources, so being prepared is the best defense.

It's best to come up with three or four responses to comments that bother you. I had a patient who was big when she was pregnant. People would walk up to her and say, "OMG, you are so big!" She'd respond, "Yes, I'm carrying ten" or "Gee, thanks a lot." You can be calm and considerate or zing them if you want. If they are being particularly intrusive, a snappy comeback can cut off the conversation. If they share horror stories, simply say, "I don't want to hear that, thank you." You can be polite but make it clear that you are not interested.

> **If they say,** "I had no nausea," **you say,** "Thank you for sharing."
> **If they say,** "I only gained eleven pounds," **you say,** "So great for you."
> **If they say,** "You must be carrying a boy, " and you know you are having a girl, **you can either smile and nod and say,** "Yup, you're right, and my doctor must be wrong," or laugh and say that all women in your family carry as if they were having boys.

Do keep a few comeback lines at the ready to get the person to back off. Sometimes people need reminding, in not the nicest way possible, that they have crossed a line.

Electronic Communication

Pregnancy truism: No one is as into your pregnancy as you are; if others are totally into it, they might begin to annoy you (see earlier section on mothers-in-law). Don't forget that you are going to be *a whole lot* more interested in the nuances of your pregnancy than anyone. Wait for other people to ask before volunteering information.

For those who want to know, e-mail and texting are great ways to communicate because they give you a chance to consider what to say before you say it. But don't hit "send" unless you have reviewed what you have written.

I encourage you to be very careful about how you communicate on social media sites like Facebook. I've had patients who post about the joy of their pregnancy and put information out there that they later regret. A good rule of thumb is this: If you'd rather not see it on the front page of the paper, don't post it. You may be ecstatic about the news, but do you really need friends of friends of friends knowing the intimate details of your pregnancy? Also, you may have friends who are single, infertile, or do not have a healthy baby; how much do you really want to crow about your situation?

Throughout your pregnancy, you will want to communicate effectively to those around you what you are thinking, feeling, and needing. Getting what you need isn't best done through whining or becoming a pregnancy diva. No matter how self-sufficient you are, there will probably come a time when you will need or want some help. If you keep your requests honest, considerate, and empathic, you will help yourself to get what you need and avoid any communication confusion.

Chapter 8

The Fourth Trimester— the Bump Is Now a Baby!

CONGRATULATIONS, THE BUMP is now a baby! Welcome to the world of parenthood. It has become common to refer to the first three months of a baby's life as the fourth trimester. You are no longer pregnant, but you (and your baby) are in a transitional phase where your life can shift from feeling magical to overwhelmed in seconds and then right back again. This chapter will give you some ideas and support on how to make the adjustment from pregnancy to life with baby.

Life after pregnancy can have emotional highs and lows. It's hard, but it has the potential to be really great. Some of it is up to your baby, and some of it is up to you. The goal of this chapter is to help you to get your needs met so that you can have that magical mommy/baby time you dreamed of.

You may be more tired than you have ever been in your

life, especially if you are breast-feeding. If you had trouble sleeping during pregnancy, you might have become used to functioning with less sleep than you would like. Pregnancy has a way of doing that—preparing you for what is to come. Trust me, you are going to feel okay again, and you will get your body back. You just need to be patient and stop reading those body-after-baby articles in magazines. And remember, many celebrities these days are using surrogates to carry their babies, so getting their body back after baby is simply a matter of taking off the fake-baby-bump pillow.

The first few days and weeks of having your baby home are a time for you all to get used to one another and figure out what works best for each of you. Babies grow and change pretty quickly, so if one day you find yourself thinking, "OMG, I can't do this *forever*," know that you won't have to. Think about what you can do today—what you can do today for yourself and what you need to do today for your baby. That is the same advice I gave during pregnancy. I advised you not to focus on getting through the first trimester but to focus on getting through that one day when you felt yucky. Same goes for your baby today. Just because he didn't sleep much last night does not mean he won't sleep tonight. Take it one day at a time. Every day.

One thing you have to adapt to is the constant needs of your newborn. When your baby was in utero, it was protected, and your body did all the baby care automatically. Your job was to eat well and rest when possible. Now that the baby is out in the world, however, you need to be vigilant and keep him warm, dry, fed, and amused—which can feel a little (or a lot) overwhelming. However, if you over-dramatize, you will find yourself in *always* and *never* land. The baby *always* cries. I will *never* get to sleep. Remember the technique in chapter 4 for testing the truth of statements? Well, it applies here too.

Here's an example.

You: The baby was up every two hours last night, and I am exhausted from getting up with her. I can't do this. It's too hard. I am too tired. She is clearly a terrible sleeper, she will always be an awful sleeper, and I am never, ever going to get a good night's rest.

Reframed You: Wow, last night was awful. I don't know what was going on with the baby. I need to take charge and figure out how to get more sleep. I have to remind myself that sleep issues tend to go away with time, that there are things I can do to get more sleep such as giving her a bottle of formula late at night so she sleeps better, or pumping during the day so my partner can feed her a couple of times during the night. I am really tired right now but know that this is not the way I will always feel.

One thing that frustrates new moms is their inability to get things accomplished. Someone who used to work full-time, maintain a nice home, and still have time for family and friends suddenly isn't able to shower on a daily basis. I remember when my first daughter, Sarah, was about six weeks old, my husband, Dave, came home from work and cheerfully asked me what I had accomplished that day. I told him that I had emptied the dishwasher. He laughed, and said, "Seriously, what did you get done today?" It is amazing that he survived that comment. But despite how difficult that day was—when I was convinced that I would be nursing that baby the rest of my life—in a blink of an eye my kids were emptying the dishwasher.

Co-parenting with Your Partner

You two are in this together, and while the divisions of labor (especially if you are breast-feeding) may fall more squarely on your shoulders, don't forget that your partner should play a significant role too. Keep in mind, however, that you and your partner may not take care of the baby in the exact same way. He may do everything differently from you, and that's okay. Don't be the know-it-all and correct his efforts—unless it's over a safety issue.

You really don't want your partner to give you all the responsibility all the time. It's nice to feel indispensable, but resist the urge! If you are the only one who can get the baby to sleep, the only one who can get him changed or bathed or any of the myriad things a baby needs, you will have a tough time down the road. You are setting yourself up to be the sole caretaker, and the baby is getting used to the way you do things. With a variety of people caring for her, she won't only respond to one way of doing things. It's important to share the responsibility and not assume that you are the expert and that your partner knows nothing. Different doesn't mean wrong or bad. As long as the basics are met—support the baby's head, change those dirty diapers, feed, burp, and get her to sleep—the baby is going to be just fine. In addition, it's important for you to have breaks to rest and recharge. It can feel as if the whole world revolves around your baby (and for a time it does), but you need to be back in the world yourself and see friends and engage in the activities you enjoyed before baby.

Getting the Help You Need

Many women receive an outpouring of offers to help when they have a baby. If people ask, "Can I help?" you should say, "Yes!" Here is a great way to take them up on the offer—even if there isn't something you need right the minute that they ask: Whenever people offer to help, write down their names and contact information. Then, when you need something, go down the list and figure out whom you can call on to help. Does your neighbor love your dog? Ask him to take the dog for a walk if you are pressed for time with the baby. Is your best friend an amazing cook? Next time she visits, ask if she could bring that yummy casserole she makes so you can freeze it for a future meal. Have your mom help with the birth announcements, or ask your mother-in-law if she can pick up the stroller you ordered. When you are out of diapers and are too tired to drive, call and ask someone if she can do it for you. You can't do it all, and if you are up every two hours to nurse, you may be too tired to think clearly. People want to help, and if you ask for what you really need, and ask nicely, you'll be in great shape.

It's also a great idea to make use of resources that may be available to you in your neighborhood or town. Your number one resource is other moms. There is salvation in shared misery. Check your local LISTSERV for mom support groups. Ask your pediatrician about any local parenting or new-baby groups. Find those other moms out there, and start a playgroup of your own. (Frankly, a playgroup for infants is really for the moms, and it's a great opportunity to share stories, commiserate over lack of sleep, and exchange ideas for coping with everything from feeding to sex issues.) Meet up with someone from your childbirth class. Sometimes religious institutions offer spaces to mother-and-child groups, so ask at the local preschool if they know of any groups. If you have friends or neighbors with babies or small children, you can pool your resources and offer to watch each other's children so one of you can run errands or even take a nap.

Centuries ago, women had a network of family and neighbors that kicked in automatically when a baby was born. Now it takes more of an effort to find a community and build a network of support, but it is definitely worth it!

Sleep Solutions

Babies aren't great sleepers at first. It's inevitable that your sleep will be affected by when, how, and if your baby sleeps. I tell my patients to nap any chance they can take. The baby is going to be okay sleeping while you nap; *you* need to sleep. Or ask someone to come over to watch the baby so you can sleep. My mother used to come over several afternoons per week for months after the birth of my first daughter. My daughter was not a happy napper (for me anyway), but I swear that she would take one look at my mom, sigh against her shoulder, and sleep for hours in her arms. Which meant that I could crash on my bed and get some much-needed sleep or even just rest. It can be difficult to nap if you are not used to it (particularly during the day), so using relaxation techniques can ease you into some much-needed rest. Try deep breathing; do mini relaxations until you get drowsy (see appendix I).

Take a deep breath. Try breathing in with your nose and out with your mouth. As you inhale, focus on the coolness of the air you breathe in. As you exhale, focus on the warmth. You can even say "cool" to yourself as you inhale and "warm" to yourself as you exhale.

One of the biggest triggers for depression during pregnancy and postpartum is sleep deprivation. You *need* to find a way to get more sleep. If you are breast-feeding, you can pump, and your partner can do some feedings so you don't have to wake up in the night and can sleep through a couple of feedings. Or you can use formula at night so your partner can feed the baby. Partners can also suffer during the postpartum period with insomnia and lack of sleep. Find a way to help each other through this period. Taking turns works well. So, for example, you go to bed at 9:00 p.m., he does the 11:00 p.m. feeding, you do the 1:00 a.m., which means you have had four hours of sleep, then he does the 3:00 a.m., and so on. I think that system works better than taking turns for entire nights, but try each method and see which works better for the two of you.

You will soon learn your baby's rhythms and behaviors. Sometimes babies can fuss and move around while sleeping but then can get themselves back to sleep. I recommend not getting up unless the baby is really crying. It's hard to resist the urge, but if you rush in at the slightest sound, the baby won't learn to calm himself. Use a baby monitor so you can keep tabs on whether or not your baby really needs you to come and soothe him back to sleep.

Emotions

Just about any emotion you experience after giving birth is normal and to be expected. Feeling overwhelmed, anxious, and angry at your partner, as well as feeling super happy or crying for joy, can all occur at this time. And sometimes at the same time! It is also normal to worry that something will happen to you or your partner. When I went back to work from maternity leave after the birth of my first daughter, a new mother came in with the complaint that she was suddenly super worried about her own health. My response? Wow, me too! You have to figure that when your therapist has the same issue as you, it has to be normal, right? This is the time when many new parents come face-to-face with their own fears about mortality. It's hard not to when this helpless little being is your world.

Common Thoughts

Volatility of emotions is to be expected in the postpartum period. You can have minute-to-minute changes in the way you are feeling.

I'm so happy!

What was I thinking?

I'll never sleep again!

I love breast-feeding!

I hate breast-feeding!

I cry at everything.

I have no idea what I'm doing.

I love being a mom.

I'm worried that I'm a terrible mom.

Sometimes I resent all that the baby needs from me.

I love that my baby needs me.

The Baby Blues and Postpartum Depression

If you have any history of depression and anxiety, your antennae need to be up for postpartum depression. Postpartum is being talked about more these days, and there is less stigma attached to it. I think that Brooke Shields has done so much good by going public with her own struggles. Any time a celebrity talks honestly about her own health issue, it takes some of the stigma away and makes society so much more aware of the problem.

Alert your partner or those you spend time with to what you are feeling and thinking. You can't ignore postpartum depression. There are many options for treating it, including CBT, exercise, and medication. Depression doesn't only affect you; it can have an effect on your baby as well. Women who are depressed tend to interact less with their infants and are less attuned to their baby's needs. If you treat your depressive symptoms, not only will you feel better, but your baby will be better off as well.

If you feel more depressed than the simple baby blues, it is very important to talk to someone right away. Talk to a friend, talk to your partner, talk to your OB, talk to your therapist. The best thing you can do for yourself and your baby is to get the support you need.

Baby Blues—can last a few days or weeks:[1]

- "One minute I'm happy, and the next I'm upset."
- "I worry, worry, worry."
- "I feel sad."
- "I snap at people and feel on edge."
- "I cry at the drop of a hat."
- "I'm distracted."
- "I'm tired, but I can't seem to get to sleep or stay asleep."

Postpartum Depression
(one in five mothers suffer from postpartum depression).[2]
Symptoms are more severe or intense than the
baby blues and can last for months:

- "I don't feel like eating."
- "I can't sleep."
- "I'm super angry about small things."
- "I'm exhausted."
- "Sex doesn't interest me."
- "I can't seem to find joy in my life."
- "I feel useless and worthless."
- "My mood seems to change every minute from one extreme to another."
- "I don't feel connected with my baby."
- "I don't want to see anyone or be with family or friends."
- "I've thought about hurting myself or my baby."

Although Brittany experienced depression during both her pregnancies and postpartum after her second, she had great support from her partner: "He was tuned in to how I was feeling. He pointed out when I wasn't feeling great. He suggested I seek professional help before my doctor did." She went on Zoloft to deal with her postpartum depression, and it helped her to get through this period.

Some emotions can be unpleasant but are to be expected.

It is only if you have unrelenting concerns about hurting yourself or your baby that you must speak with someone immediately. If you have thoughts that won't go away, which include hurting your baby or yourself, you need to call your obstetrician right away. If you can't reach him or her, go straight to the emergency room or call 911. You might be having a very rare postpartum psychosis, which can be treated quickly and effectively, but it has to be in a hospital setting. Symptoms of postpartum psychosis include the following:[3]

- disorientation/confusion
- hallucinations/delusions
- paranoia
- attempts or plans to harm self or baby

Getting to Sleep

As mentioned previously, lack of sleep can be a huge trigger for depression and anxiety. So it's important to prioritize getting enough rest. Sleeping like a baby is an expression that doesn't have much relevance for many new parents. Babies can wake up every hour or two, sleep only when held, or sleep only in your bed. My second child had her days and nights switched so she slept soundly throughout the day and was awake much of the night. I had a four-year-old to take care of, so I couldn't simply adapt to the baby's schedule. When I was going through this, I found that walks did more for me to clear my head than taking naps. If you can't sleep, exercise can do a lot for you.

Think back to what worked for you when you were tired, anxious, or depressed during your pregnancy. If it worked when you were pregnant, it will likely work for you now that you have a baby.

Medication and Breast-Feeding

Ask your OB or nurse-midwife for a list of medications you should not take while breast-feeding. Some medications that you shouldn't take during pregnancy are okay to take when you are breast-feeding. Some women who are on medication for depression, anxiety, or other mood disorders take a break during pregnancy and then go back on the medication once the baby is born, and formula feed. If you find that you can't function without your medication and it's not recommended to breast-feed while taking it, you are probably better off formula feeding. Yes, there are benefits to breast-feeding, but if taking the medication allows you to be a fully engaged and healthy mom, then the trade-offs are worth it.

There is some controversy over whether SSRIs (antidepressants) are okay to take when you are breast-feeding.

SSRIs may cross over into your milk, so I'm not all that comfortable with saying it's okay to take SSRIs while breastfeeding. Talk to your doctor. You can try cognitive behavioral therapy or other therapies before going on medications when you are nursing. However, if you are a risk to anyone (yourself or your baby), medication is likely your best option.

Transitioning Back to Work

The when and how of going back to work is very dependent on your particular situation. You have to weigh the pros and cons financially (that is, can you afford to stay home?), emotionally, and practically. To determine the best situation for you, you need to discuss with your partner what will work best for your family. Some women return to work, some work part-time after the baby is born, and some stay home full-time. One woman said that going back to work was a big point of contention between herself and her husband. "He likes the identity I have when I work full-time," she said, "but right now that's not my number one identity."

Holly, who is twenty-four weeks pregnant, is concerned about going back to work. "Trying to figure out how to work after pregnancy is stressful and makes me anxious. I'm dreading having to think about it."

For Melissa, who has one child and is thirty-three weeks

pregnant with her second, the choice about work isn't so easy. "Everyone talks about the choices women have to make, and I never really understood it until now. I'm a big analyzer, so I talk with my husband, mom, and friends. Before I had kids, I thought I'd know, either way, what was right for me. But I'm ambivalent, and it feels like a roller coaster."

If you plan to return to work after maternity leave ("the average maternity leave in the U.S. is about 10 weeks, but about half of new moms took at least five weeks, with about a quarter taking nine weeks or more"[4]), it can help if you have kept up with work while you were out; checking e-mail, touching base with the office, and occasionally going in to meetings will help you not feel slammed or out of the loop when you return. You don't want to feel as if you've missed out on everything at the office while you've been home with your baby. During my second maternity leave, I took my baby with me to an important meeting, and when she got fussy, I began to nurse her, figuring that everyone else in the room was either a doctor or a nurse and wouldn't be fazed. My boss, a physician but of an older generation, ran the entire meeting with his back turned! The following week I brought a bottle.

It's a good idea to line up child care in advance of your return to work. You want to be able to get to know your caregiver or be familiar with the child-care or day-care center before you leave your baby for a full workday. This is another situation where you want to tap into your mom network for information and resources. Your pediatrician may also know of potential caregivers or centers.

Beyond the Fourth Trimester

Being a mom is only *one* of your roles. As wonderful as your baby is, don't make your baby your whole world. Your job is to do all you can so that, someday, your baby can be independent of you. Let other people hold, take care of, and love your baby. Babies need to be around other people, get some fresh air, and experience the world. You are going to have doubts; you are not going to be the perfect mother. You will make mistakes, but children are astoundingly resilient, and the two of you will grow and learn together.

Notes

Chapter 2: Pregnancy Perfection

1. University of Missouri-Columbia, "If Facebook Causes Envy, Depression Could Follow," *ScienceDaily*, Feb. 3, 2015.
2. Penn State, "Expectant Moms Turn to Internet for Pregnancy Advice More than They Would Like," *ScienceDaily*, July 7, 2014.

Chapter 3: Pregnancy Survival Kit

1. Tara Parker-Pope, "Writing Your Way to Happiness," *Well* (blog), *The New York Times*, Jan. 19, 2015.
2. Alice D. Domar et al., "The Risks of Selective Serotonin Reuptake Inhibitor Use in Infertile Women: A Review of the Impact on Fertility, Pregnancy, Neonatal Health, and

Beyond," *Human Reproduction* 28, no. 1 (2013): 160–71, doi: 10.1093/humrep/des383.

3. University of Michigan Health System, "Walking Off Depression and Beating Stress Outdoors? Nature Group Walks Linked to Improved Mental Health," *ScienceDaily*, Sept. 23, 2014.

4. Cooper WO, Willy ME, Pont SJ, et al., "Increasing Use of Antidepressants in Pregnancy," *Am J Obstet Gynecol* 2007: 196.

5. Anahad O'Connor, "New York Attorney General Targets Supplements at Major Retailers," *The New York Times*, Feb. 3, 2015.

Chapter 4: The Pregnant Brain

1. Massachusetts General Hospital Center for Women's Mental Health, "Psychiatric Disorders During Pregnancy," http://womensmentalhealth.org/specialty -clinics/psychiatric-disorders-during-pregnancy/.

Chapter 5: High-Octane Prenatal Self-Care

1. American Congress of Obstetricians and Gynecologists, "WEBTREATS: Diet, Weight Management, and Obesity," www.acog.org/About-ACOG/ACOG -Departments/Resource-Center/WEBTREATS -Diet-Weight-Mgmt-Obesity.

2. Recipe for Food Safety, www.cdc.gov/vitalsigns/listeria/.

3. Karolinska Institutet, "How Physical Exercise Protects the Brain from Stress-Induced Depression," *ScienceDaily*, Sept. 25, 2014.

Chapter 6: Belly Support

1. U.S. Department of Labor, Wage and Hour Division, Family and Medical Leave Act, www.dol.gov/whd/fmla/.

Chapter 7: Talking Your Way Through Pregnancy

1. U.S. Department of Labor, Wage and Hour Division, Family and Medical Leave Act, www.dot.gov/whd/fmla/.

2. Adam Liptak, "UPS Suit Hinges on an Ambiguous Pregnancy Law," *The New York Times*, Dec. 3, 2014.

3. Elizabeth Armstrong Moore, "Suit: Pregnant Woman Fired over Bathroom Breaks," *USA Today*, Dec. 5, 2014.

Chapter 8: The Fourth Trimester—the Bump Is Now a Baby!

1. Mayo Clinic Staff, Postpartum Depression, www.mayoclinic.org/diseases-conditions/postpartum-depression/basics/symptoms/con-20029130.

2. Shoshana S. Bennett and Pec Indman, *Beyond the Blues: A Guide to Understanding and Treating Prenatal and Postpartum Depression* (San Jose: Moodswings Press, 2006).

3. Mayo Clinic Staff, Postpartum Depression.

4. JoNel Aleccia, "Two Weeks After Baby? More New Moms Cut Maternity Leave Short," *Today*, Sept. 27, 2013, www.today.com.

Acknowledgments

Many authors describe their books as their "babies." Unlike a baby who needs two parents to create it, this book has had far more than just Sheila and me as parents. I would like to thank Alice Lesch Kelly, who helped me come up with the concept of this book and co-wrote the proposal. Wendy Sherman, my agent, was sort of like an obstetrician, congratulating me on the conception of the book, hovering nearby if needed, but allowing me to labor at my own pace. I also want to thank my niece Rachel Domar Banderob for coming up with the title of the book.

I will forever owe my interest in creating books to Henry Dreher and Chris Tomasino. Our first "baby" is now twenty. The time has flown by, and Henry just passed away, tragically, far too soon, but my gratitude to him for holding my hand as we wrote *Healing Mind, Healthy Woman* together and to you, Chris, for believing in me so long ago.

I want to thank Theresa Raso and Robin Laskey, who together keep the Domar Center up and running; it is not only a wonderful resource for patients but a pleasure to work in. My colleagues at Boston IVF are continually supportive of all of my clinical and writing endeavors, for which I am eternally grateful. Adam Urato, MD, through an initial lecture followed by a long collaboration, introduced me to the research on the risks of antidepressant medication during pregnancy and has been supportive and gracefully informative throughout the creation of this book.

I will always be grateful to my patients who trust in me to help them, who agree to be included in my books, and who make me love coming to work every day. And to all the pregnant women who agreed to be interviewed for this book, thank you. I know that talking about physical and emotional discomfort during pregnancy with a perfect stranger wasn't at the top of your to-do list, but your willingness to share has made this a richer guide for others.

I would also like to acknowledge my writer, Sheila. We literally met while halfway through the book, and my hat is off to you. You agreed to do this after one phone call and had no idea how zany a person I truly am. Thank you for your patience, your humor, and your empathy. I loved talking with you. I truly think you should be a therapist in your next life.

And finally, my love and appreciation to my family. To my husband, Dave, who not only tolerated with wonderful humor my complaining and moaning through two pregnancies but has taken over the laundry and numerous other household chores to allow me time to work on this book and has been supportive of my career 100 percent of the time. And to my girls, Sarah and Katie, you have shown me that pregnancy is truly worth it and that having a baby is just the beginning of the best adventure of life.

The Calm Mom-to-Be

Mind/Body Techniques
to Reduce Stress and Anxiety

Following are some of the mind/body techniques that have appeared throughout the book. This is essentially a tool kit for you to use while you are pregnant. These techniques can also come in handy for when your bump is born. Mind/body techniques are great in that they can be used when you are faced with any challenge and need to tap into your inner resources to overcome what you are experiencing.

Write It Out

Getting down on paper what you think and feel can be very beneficial. It can allow you time to review and reflect and, hopefully, come to a better understanding of your situation.

Our minds can race at a mile a minute, so slowing down to write can help you to see things in a different light. The next time you are sad, angry, or upset, sit down with pen and paper and write down what is going on to make you feel the way you do. There is no need to save what you have written if you don't want to, but sometimes getting it on paper and rereading it at a later date can give you a fresh perspective. The key is to write about your thoughts and feelings, rather than simply reciting what happened.

Mindfulness

Mindfulness can be brought to nearly any activity or situation—eating or walking, for example. When you are engaged mindfully, you can ask yourself the following questions:

- What do I hear?
- What do I feel?
- What do I smell?
- What do I see?
- What do I taste (if eating)?

By taking the time to ask these questions and thoughtfully respond, you allow yourself to be more fully engaged in the activity and deepen your experience. It will also allow you to take a break from what's going on in your head and with your emotions because you will bring your focus to your mindful activity and away from any negative chatter that is bringing you down. I found breast-feeding mindfully to be wonderfully relaxing.

Self-Nurturance

A favorite phrase of someone I know is "If you don't ask, you don't get." In the case of taking care of yourself, you need to stop and think about what you need. You have the ability to define not only what you need but how to get it.

When you are faced with fear, sadness, or any discomfort, ask yourself, "What will make me feel

... *Happier?"*
... *Healthier?"*
... *More energetic?"*

You may be able to help yourself feel better, or you may need to seek assistance from your partner, friends, family, or therapist. Until you ask for help, you won't know how much easier it can get.

Getting the Support You Need

It's rare that any of us takes the time to stop and think, "What do I need?" Take the time now to ask yourself this question. Stop and think about things like *What makes me feel better? What makes me feel worse?* Once you have recognized your needs (*what makes me feel better*), as well as the things you need to eliminate from your life, even temporarily (*what makes me feel worse*), figure out who in your life can meet them. Partner? Other family members? Co-worker? Friend? Church? Self? Then ask, nicely, for what you need their help with.

Couples' Communication

There will be times when you and your partner may be in conflict over a situation or issue. And while it is tempting to get angry, you can get a lot more communicated and accomplished by using the basic formula for couples' communication:

It makes me feel _____ when you _____

because _____.

Cognitive Restructuring

There is a very simple technique that can help you to rein in those runaway thoughts and cut your catastrophic thinking down to size. It requires writing and reflecting on the thought, so you might want to keep a pen and small notebook by the side of your bed so you can write down the intrusive thought, promise yourself that you will tackle it in the morning, and get back to your much-needed sleep. You can do the same thing in the light of day. Monitor your repetitive thoughts, jot them down, and tackle them when you have a few minutes for reflection.

The Four Questions

First, write down the thought. Then ask yourself the following questions:

1. Does this thought contribute to my stress?
2. Where did I learn this thought? These thoughts usually come from something someone said to you in the past, or it is your fear speaking.
3. Is this a logical thought?
4. Is this thought true?

Once you have evaluated your thought for truth and logic, you can restructure it so that the emotional aspect has been removed and it has become a true and logical statement.

Stop, Breathe, Reflect, and Choose

When an intrusive or negative thought pops up:

Stop—Visualize a stop sign.

Breathe—Slow down, take a few slow breaths.

Reflect—Ask, "What is really going on here?"

Choose—Make the choice to do something that you know will make you feel better. Try to restructure the thought, reframe the idea, take a walk, talk to your partner, have a cup of tea, or call the doctor. Knowing you have a choice increases your sense of control and will make you feel less anxious.

Be Prepared and Reduce Anxiety

When you are faced with a pregnancy-related issue, come up with a strategy that will help you address the problem, and put the plan in place. Make a list of issues, their triggers, and their antidotes.

Issue: _____

_____

Trigger: _____

_____

Antidote: _____

_____

Mini Relaxation Techniques

Being with Baby

Sit comfortably with your hands on your belly or in your lap. For a few minutes, just sit and be with your baby; feel it move inside you. Take a little time to experience the miracle that you are creating.

A Good Breath of Calming Air
(The Mini Relaxation)

Close your eyes, and take a couple of slow, deep breaths. Say the number "ten" to yourself as you inhale, and then slowly exhale. For the next breath, say the number "nine" to yourself, and then slowly exhale. Do this until you get down to zero. Try opening your eyes. Feel any more relaxed?

Or, as you take slow comfortable breaths, count from one to four as you inhale, and then count from four to one as you exhale. Do that five times.

Following Your Breath

Much like "A Good Breath of Calming Air," this exercise helps you to carve out some calm in your day and to allow your breathing to come evenly and deeply. (Have you ever noticed that when you are tense, your breathing seems to increase and gets shallow?) Sitting comfortably, gently close your eyes, let your shoulders drop, and inhale a deep breath through your nose, hold it for a count of three, and let it go out of your mouth until you feel empty, then hold it for another count of three. Then fill up through your nose again, and repeat the process. Visualize good, calm air coming in through your nose, and see "bad" anxious air filled with negative thoughts leave you as you exhale.

Eliciting the Relaxation Response

The relaxation response is a general description of the changes that occur in your body when you use any of a variety of relaxation techniques. These techniques include meditation, yoga, progressive muscle relaxation, imagery, autogenic training, and breath focus. They allow you to take some time out of your day to rest and recharge. While you elicit the relaxation response, you will likely feel calmer and more relaxed, even for a few moments. If you make a habit of it, you will began to feel the benefits throughout the day, not just while you are focusing on a technique.

Sitting and focusing your mind on your breath, body, or a repetitive phrase doesn't seem like much, but it can have a profound effect on your mind and mood when you make it a habit. First, select a comfortable chair (not too comfortable or you might find yourself dozing off); next, simply sit. It's best to sit for at least twenty minutes, but do what you can. It is also beneficial to do your relaxation technique at the same time and place every day; carve out the time for yourself by writing in your calendar and letting your partner know you need a few minutes alone at this time each day.

Meditation

Meditation is a wonderful way to relieve stress. The basic goal is to quiet the mind and to let go of any thoughts that are troubling you. The key is to focus on a word or phrase and repeat it silently to yourself in rhythm with your breath. Meditating for even a few minutes can be beneficial. Sit comfortably in a chair with your feet firmly on the floor. Allow your hands to rest in your lap (or, depending on how big your bump is, rest gently on your bump). Close your eyes and breathe normally. The more you do it, the less your mind will wander.

If the phrase you're meditating on is, for example, "breathing in peace and calm," say half the phrase to yourself as you inhale and the other half as you exhale. When I was pregnant with my first daughter, Sarah, I began to have premature contractions and was restricted to bed rest. Her due date was January 30. I would meditate daily and say on my inhalation, "I will make it," and on the exhalation, "to January." She was born January 9!

If a thought comes up, acknowledge it, but don't start chasing it down. See it in your mind's eye, and let it go. It's almost as if you were gently turning the thought away. When you have been sitting for a few minutes, open your eyes, stand up, stretch, and continue with your day.

Relaxation Techniques That
Are Especially Good for Getting to Sleep

The Body Scan is a way to seek out parts of your body that may be holding tension that needs to be released in order for you to relax into sleep and get the rest you need.

Lie on your bed, in as comfortable a position as you can find, your hands at your sides, palms up. Breathe gently and evenly. Allow your belly to rise with each breath (not your chest). Starting with your forehead, work your way down through all of your body parts, pausing to see if you can identify any tension or pain. Relax the tension in that body part by focusing your breath there and letting the tension go. By the time you get to your toes, you should be ready to drift off to sleep. So, for example, you start by focusing on your forehead. As you inhale, focus all your attention on your forehead, and as you exhale, concentrate on relaxing your forehead muscles. Then move down to the muscles around your eyes, your cheeks, your lower jaw, and so on.

Progressive Muscle Relaxation is very similar to the body scan except that you take a more active role in releasing any tension in a particular body part. Lie comfortably on your bed, hands at sides, palms up. To begin, breathe deeply and gently, allowing your belly to rise with each breath. Then, starting with your forehead, squeeze those muscles tight and hold for a count of five, then release. Next, squeeze your eyes tight, hold for a count of five, and release. Progress through your body and muscle groups. Pay attention to any areas where you typically feel muscle tension and fatigue.

Options for Healing

These approaches can help you to self-nurture, relax, safely express your emotions, and let go of perfectionism. If you take a group class, you can gain some social support from either an instructor who understands what you are going through or other pregnant women who may be experiencing physical and emotional symptoms similar to yours.

Acupuncture—If you choose acupuncture, be sure the practitioner is knowledgeable about treating a pregnant woman. Acupuncture is safe to use during pregnancy and is an effective treatment for nausea/vomiting, as well as depression and anxiety.

Exercise—As I have said before, exercise will do more for you than anything else. It is a happy pill that's free and has no side effects. If you stay fit, you can decrease anxiety and depression and feel more in control. But make sure your obstetrician or nurse-midwife is comfortable with your exercise regimen.

Light Therapy—Exposure to particular light waves can serve to elevate mood. This therapy is often used for people who have seasonal affective disorder. A box emits light that is similar to sunlight, countering its lack in fall and winter, when SAD is most likely to occur. There is a potential for light therapy to trigger mania in those with bipolar disorder, so please check with your doctor first.

Massage—Massage is wonderful for relieving aches and pains, but when you are pregnant, be sure to get a massage from someone who is familiar with working with pregnant women and is skilled in prenatal massage.

Supplements—Women are advised to take a prenatal vitamin prior to getting pregnant (if possible) and then throughout the pregnancy. There are hundreds of other supplements available in your grocery store, health food store, local pharmacy, and online. Please be careful about what you take. Ask your OB or nurse-midwife before taking any supplement other than a prenatal vitamin.

Yoga—There are many forms of yoga, and prenatal yoga classes (taught by an experienced instructor) can give you a gentle workout and allow you to turn off your mind for a little while. Many of my patients love going to a prenatal yoga class because it gives them a chance to partake in an effective relaxation technique and keep fit while also providing social support during the time spent with other pregnant women.

Appendix II

Resources

Bookshelf—Recommended Reading from Other Moms

The Boston Women's Health Book Collective. *Our Bodies, Ourselves: Pregnancy and Birth*. New York: Touchstone, 2008.

DK Publishing and Maggie Blott. *Pregnancy Day By Day*. New York: Dorling Kindersley, 2013.

England, Pam, and Rob Horowitz. *Birthing from Within: An Extra-Ordinary Guide to Childbirth Preparation*. Albuquerque: Partera Press, 1998.

Farber, Elaine. *Baby Lists: What to Do and What to Get to Prepare for Baby*. Avon, MA: Adams Media, 2007.

Gaskin, Ina May. *Ina May's Guide to Childbirth*. New York: Bantam, 2003.

Hakakha, Michele, and Ari Brown. *Expecting 411: The Insider's Guide to Pregnancy and Childbirth, 3rd ed.* Boulder: Windsor Peak Press, 2014.

Karp, Harvey. *The Happiest Baby on the Block.* New York: Bantam, 2003.

Magee, Susan, and Kara Nakisbendi. *The Pregnancy Countdown Book: Nine Months of Practical Tips, Useful Advice, and Uncensored Truths.* Philadelphia: Quirk Books, 2012.

McCarthy, Jenny. *Belly Laughs: The Naked Truth about Pregnancy and Childbirth, 10th Anniversary Ed.* Cambridge, MA: Da Capo Press, 2014.

Murkoff, Heidi, and Sharon Mazel. *What to Expect When You're Expecting.* New York: Workman, 2008.

Odes, Rebecca, and Ceridwen Morris. *From the Hips: A Comprehensive, Open-Minded, Uncensored, Totally Honest Guide to Pregnancy, Birth, and Becoming a Parent.* New York: Harmony, 2007.

Oster, Emily. *Expecting Better: Why the Conventional Pregnancy Wisdom Is Wrong and What You Really Need to Know.* New York: Penguin Books, 2014.

Verrilli, George, and Anne Marie Mueser. *While Waiting.* New York: St. Martin's Press, 2002.

Additional Recommended Reading

Burns, David D. *The Feeling Good Handbook*. New York: Plume, 1999.

Pennebaker, James, and John Evans. *Expressive Writing: Words that Heal*. Enumclaw, WA: Idyll Arbor, 2014.

Wilson, Timothy D. *Redirect: Changing the Stories We Live By*. New York: Back Bay, 2015.

Web Sites That Are Typically Reliable

American Academy of Pediatrics	www.aap.org
American Congress of Obstetricians and Gynecologists	www.acog.org
American Heart Association	www.heart.org
Centers for Disease Control and Prevention	www.cdc.gov
Family and Medical Leave Act	www.dol.gov/whd/fmla/
Marcé Society for Perinatal Mental Health	https://marcesociety.com

North American Society for Psychosocial Obstetrics and Gynecology — www.naspog.org

Postpartum Support International — www.postpartum.net

WebMD — www.webmd.com

Apps and Commercial Web Sites

Baby Center — www.babycenter.com
The Bump — www.thebump.com
Lucie's list — www.lucieslist.com
Ovia (app) — www.ovuline.com
Pregnancy + (app) — https://itunes.apple.com/us/app/pregnancy-+/id505864483?mt=8

Index

About the Author

Alice D. Domar, PhD, is a pioneer in the application of mind/body medicine to women's health issues. She not only established the first Mind/Body Center for Women's Health but also conducts groundbreaking research in the field. Her research focuses on the relationship between stress and different women's health conditions, and she has created many innovative programs to help women decrease physical and psychological symptoms.

Dr. Domar was also the series editor for a series of mind/body books by Harvard Health Publications/Simon & Schuster. She is the narrator of the DVDs *Stress and Relaxation Explained* and *Infertility Explained*, both of which won silver Telly Awards.

A seasoned media authority and go-to guest, Dr. Domar has appeared on *Today*, *Good Morning America*, *CBS This*

Morning, Dateline NBC, CNN, PBS, *CBS Evening News,* and *NBC Nightly News,* to name a few. She is on the advisory boards for *Shape* magazine, *Parents* magazine, and Resolve. She is on the board of experts for Sharecare.com and was a columnist for *Redbook* and *Health* magazines. She was also a featured expert on the online social health network BeWell.com.

As a much-sought-after public speaker, Dr. Domar presents lectures and conducts workshops throughout the United States and around the world and went on tour with Oprah in the spring of 2004 and 2005 with the LLuminari team. Dr. Domar was named in the prestigious list of 15 "Women to Watch in 2004" by Lifetime TV and "100 Women to Watch in Wellness" by MindBodyGreen in 2015.

Dr. Domar received her MA and PhD in health psychology from Albert Einstein College of Medicine/Ferkauf School of Professional Psychology of Yeshiva University. Her postdoctoral training was at Beth Israel Hospital, Deaconess Hospital, and Children's Hospital, all in Boston.

She has conducted research on infertility, breast cancer, menopausal symptoms, ovarian cancer, pregnancy, and premenstrual syndrome. Dr. Domar has earned an international reputation as one of the country's top women's health experts.

She is currently the executive director of the Domar Centers for Mind/Body Health and the director of integrative care services at Boston IVF. She is an associate clinical professor of obstetrics, gynecology, and reproductive biology, part-time, at Harvard Medical School and a senior staff psychologist at Beth Israel Deaconess Medical Center.

Please visit her Web sites at www.domarcenter.com and www.dralicedomar.com.

If you enjoyed this book, visit

www.tarcherperigee.com

and sign up for TarcherPerigee's e-newsletter to receive special offers, updates on hot new releases, and articles containing the information you need to live the life you want.

tarcherperigee

LEARN. CREATE. GROW.

Connect with the TarcherPerigee Community

. . .

Stay in touch with favorite authors

Enter giveaway promotions

Read exclusive excerpts

Voice your opinions

Follow us

 f TarcherPerigee

𝕏 @TarcherPerigee

⧉ @TarcherPerigee

If you would like to place a bulk order of this book,
call 1-800-733-3000.

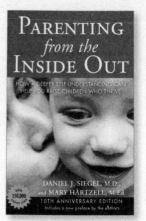
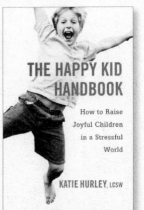
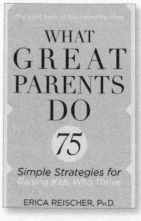